Handy Tips to Reduce the GL

- Eat small or moderate portions of starchy foods such as bread, potatoes, pasta, and rice.

- Include lots of low-GL fruit and vegetables at every meal. Aim for a minimum of five servings of fruit and veg per day. Lightly cook veggies for the minimum time or eat them raw. Fresh, frozen, or canned fruit and veg are all fine. Head to Chapter 3 for more.

- Make more of pulses including peas, beans, and lentils in soups, salads, and as a meal accompaniment instead of pasta or rice. Pulses, including dried or canned, count towards your five-a-day fruit and veg.

- Always include a protein-rich food as part of your meal to reduce the GL. Choose from lean meat, fish, poultry, eggs, low-fat dairy foods, soya products, or quorn.

- Adding acidic foods such as balsamic vinegar, lemon juice, vinaigrette, or pickles (for example, capers and gherkins) to your meal reduces the overall GL. Adding a little monounsaturated oil such as olive or rapeseed oil, or a little Parmesan cheese or reduced-fat cream to recipes also lowers the GL.

- Cut right down on highly refined snack foods such as sweets, crisps or corn chips, cakes, biscuits, and pastries made from white flour and sugar. Instead, choose nuts and seeds, or dried fruits such as apple rings or apricots. Instead of milk chocolate, snack on a couple of squares of dark chocolate with over 70 per cent cocoa solids.

Starchy Staples: Helpful Low-GL Alternatives

Starchy staple	Low GL	High GL
Bread	Pumpernickel, rye, sourdough, soya and linseed, barley and sunflower, granary, seeded breads and pitta breads (moderate GL), oat cakes, rye crackers (moderate GL)	White, wholemeal, French stick, rice cakes, cream crackers, bread sticks
Cereal	Whole oats, oatmeal, porridge, no added sugar muesli, bran sticks, semolina, quinoa	Sweetened cereals, rice based cereals, bran flakes, wheat biscuits, shredded wheat

(continued)

The GL Diet For Dummies®

Cheat Sheet

Starchy staple	Low GL	High GL
Pasta	Egg-based pasta, mungbean noodles	Overcooked pasta and pasta ready meals requiring re-heating
Rice	Long grain, wild, and basmati rice. Bulgur or cracked wheat, couscous, pearl barley	Short grain, sticky white rice
Potatoes	Baby new potatoes, sweet potatoes, yams, celeriac, swede	Large floury white potatoes, French fries, mashed potato

Low-GL Seasonal Fruit and Vegetables

	Fruits	Vegetables
Spring	Rhubarb, grapes, limes, passion fruit, sharon fruit, lemons, grapefruit, avocados	Leeks, cabbage, watercress, new potatoes, spinach, aubergines, radishes, rocket, spring greens
Summer	Strawberries, raspberries, blueberries, redcurrants, blackcurrants, cherries, nectarines, melons	Asparagus, baby carrots, fresh peas, tomatoes, runner beans, lettuce, cucumber, courgettes, peppers, mange tout
Autumn	Blackberries, apples, pears, gooseberries, damsons, plums, elderberries, greengages, plums	Pumpkin, onions, fennel, wild mushrooms, squash, turnips, red cabbage, celeriac, swede
Winter	Satsumas, clementines, cranberries, mandarins, tangerines, pears, pomegranates	Brussels sprouts, chicory, cauliflower, kale, celery, mushrooms, purple sprouting broccoli

For Dummies: Bestselling Book Series for Beginners

Praise for The GL Diet For Dummies

Macclesfield College

Learning
Resource Centre

This book is due for return on or before the last date shown below

- 8 MAY 2013

7/9/18

library@macclesfield.ac.uk
(01625) 410008

The GL Diet

FOR

DUMMIES®

by Nigel Denby and Sue Baic

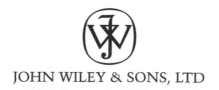

JOHN WILEY & SONS, LTD

The GL Diet For Dummies®

Published by
John Wiley & Sons, Ltd
The Atrium
Southern Gate
Chichester
West Sussex
PO19 8SQ
England

E-mail (for orders and customer service enquires): cs-books@wiley.co.uk

Visit our Home Page on www.wileyeurope.com

Wiley also publishes its books in a variety of electronic formats. Some content that appears in print may not be available in electronic books.

British Library Cataloguing in Publication Data: A catalogue record for this book is available from the British Library.

ISBN-13: 978-0-470-02753-0 (PB)

ISBN-10: 0-470-02753-3 (PB)

Printed and bound in Great Britain by TJ International, Padstow, Cornwall

10 9 8 7 6 5 4 3

WILEY

About the Authors

Nigel Denby trained as a dietitian at Glasgow Caledonian University, following an established career in the catering industry. He is also a qualified chef and previously owned his own restaurant.

His dietetic career began as a Research Dietitian at the Human Nutrition Research Centre in Newcastle upon Tyne. After a period working as a Community Dietitian, Nigel left the NHS to join Boots Health and Beauty Experience where he led the delivery and training of Nutrition and Weight Management services.

In 2003 Nigel set up his own Nutrition consultancy, delivering a clinical service to Hammersmith and Queen Charlotte's Hospital Women's Health Clinic and the International Eating Disorders Centre in Buckinghamshire as well as acting as Nutrition Consultant for the Childbase Children's Nursery Group.

Nigel also runs his own private practice in Harley Street, specialising in Weight Management, PMS / Menopause and Irritable Bowel Syndrome.

Nigel works extensively with the media, writing for the *Sunday Telegraph Magazine*, *Zest*, *Essentials*, and various other consumer magazines. His work in radio and television includes BBC and ITN news programmes, Channel 4's *Fit Farm*, BBC *Breakfast*, and BBC *Real Story*.

He is the author of *Nutrition For Dummies*.

Sue Baic is a Lecturer in Nutrition and Public Health in the Department of Exercise and Health Sciences at Bristol University. She has a first degree from Bristol University followed by a Master of Science in Human Nutrition from London University. Sue is a Registered Dietitian (RD) with over 15 years' experience in the field of nutrition and health in the NHS and as a freelance consultant. She feels strongly about providing nutrition information to the public that is evidence based, up to date, unbiased, and reliable.

As a member of the public relations committee of the British Dietetic Association she has written for the media on a variety of nutrition related health issues. Sue lives in Bristol and spends her spare time running up and down hills in the Cotswolds in an attempt to get fit.

She is the author of *Nutrition For Dummies*.

Authors' Acknowledgements

We would both like to thank the excellent team at Wiley, especially Rachael Chilvers and Alison Yates, for their part in bringing this book to fruition. Thank you too to Amelia Lake, Deborah Pyner, and Tina Michelucci for their valuable contributions.

From ND

Thanks go to my writing partner, Sue, for always spotting my typos and for her meticulous attention to detail!

From SB

Thanks to my good-natured, supportive partner, John. He, along with Rosie, helped keep me upbeat whenever deadlines were looming.

I'm also grateful to friends for their interest and encouragement with this book, and to my co-author Nigel, with whom it has been, as ever, a pleasure to work.

Publisher's Acknowledgements

We're proud of this book; please send us your comments through our Dummies online registration form located at www.dummies.com/register/.

Some of the people who helped bring this book to market include the following:

Acquisitions, Editorial, and Media Development

Development Editor: Rachael Chilvers

Content Editor: Simon Bell

Commissioning Editor: Alison Yates

Copy Editor: Juliet Booker

Proofreader: Sue Gilad

Technical Editor:
Amelia A. Lake RD, RPHNutr, PhD.
www.lakenutrition.com

Recipe Tester: Emily Nolan

Executive Editor: Jason Dunne

Executive Project Editor: Martin Tribe

Special Help: Zoë Wykes,
Jennifer Bingham

Cover Photo: © Corbis/Roy Botterell

Cartoons: Rich Tennant
(www.the5thwave.com)

Composition Services

Project Coordinators: Maridee Ennis,
Jennifer Theriot

Layout and Graphics: Joyce Haughey,
Stephanie D. Jumper, Heather Ryan,
Erin Zeltner

Proofreaders: Dwight Ramsey,
Charles Spencer, Brian Walls

Indexer: Techbooks

Publishing and Editorial for Consumer Dummies

Diane Graves Steele, Vice President and Publisher, Consumer Dummies

Joyce Pepple, Acquisitions Director, Consumer Dummies

Kristin A. Cocks, Product Development Director, Consumer Dummies

Michael Spring, Vice President and Publisher, Travel

Kelly Regan, Editorial Director, Travel

Publishing for Technology Dummies

Andy Cummings, Vice President and Publisher,
Dummies Technology/General User

Composition Services

Gerry Fahey, Vice President of Production Services

Debbie Stailey, Director of Composition Services

Contents at a Glance

Table of Contents

Introduction

*Y*ou only have to cruise the aisles of your local bookshop to find shelf upon shelf of diet books that promise staggering amount of weight loss, with minimal effort, and all achieved in the blink of an eye. What most of these 'quick fix' diet books don't tell you is that a lot of the weight you'll lose is water, sometimes you'll miss out on valuable nutrients, and what you eat is so dull, boring, and bland that you'll feel as if you're in prison rather than trying to get healthy!

The GL Diet For Dummies cuts through the diet hype and gives you an eating plan that helps you safely lose and maintain your weight for life – and boost your overall health at the same time. We don't make any empty or false promises, but we do give you heaps of tips and strategies to make the diet as easy as possible, together with delicious recipes you'll want to eat again and again. After a week or two, eating the low-GL way will feel like a way of life rather than a here today, gone tomorrow fad – that's our promise to you.

In this book we pull together everything you need to get started on a low-GL eating plan, get the results you want, and keep them forever.

About This Book

The GL Diet For Dummies doesn't give you strict rules and lists of banned foods that leave you feeling deprived and full of guilty food cravings. Instead, in this book we explain how you can stay feeling fuller for longer, experience fewer food cravings, and control your weight with an energised, healthy spring in your step. As well as being a great way to control weight, the GL Diet's best bonus is the diet is increasingly recognised as offering some real health benefits, such as lowering your risk of heart disease and diabetes.

We show you how to pick one food over another, or mix foods to lower the GL of your meal so that you're always making the best choices for your health. We also offer great tips for planning menus, food shopping, eating out, and keeping motivated on the plan.

Conventions Used in This Book

The following conventions are used throughout the text to make things consistent and easy to understand:

- All Web addresses appear in `mono font`.

- New terms appear in *italic* and are closely followed by an easy-to-understand definition.

- Both the imperial and metric measurements appear in recipes. Follow either one – just don't switch halfway through a recipe! You'll also find the American measurements. For certain ingredients known by more than one name, we put one name in brackets, such as courgette (zucchini).

- All our recipes are followed by a list that gives you the nutrient breakdown per serving.

- A little tomato symbol next to a recipe means that the meal is suitable for vegetarians. We advise you to wash your fruit and vegetables under running water before preparing them.

What You're Not to Read

You want to get to the important stuff but you're too pushed for time to read every section of every chapter? We know that feeling and so we've tried to make selecting what to take note of a bit easier for you. Some parts of this book are fun and/or informative but not necessarily vital to your understanding of GL. For example:

- **Text in sidebars:** The sidebars are the shaded boxes that appear here and there. Sidebars share anecdotes and observations but aren't essential reading.

✔ **Anything with a Technical Stuff icon attached:** This information may be interesting but is not critical to your understanding of GL.

Foolish Assumptions

Every *For Dummies* book is written with a particular reader in mind, and this one is no different. As we wrote this book, we made the following basic assumptions about who you are:

✔ You didn't study nutrition at school or university but now you've discovered that you have a better chance of staying healthy if you know how to put together a well-balanced, nutritious diet for you and your family.

✔ You're confused about which diet really is the best one to keep control of your weight and stay healthy, and you're dissatisfied with quick fixes, fads, and 'wonder diets'.

✔ You want basic information, but you don't want to become an expert in weight control and healthy eating or spend hours digging your way through medical textbooks and journals.

How This Book Is Organised

We designed this book so you don't have to start with Chapter 1 and read straight through to the end. You can dive in absolutely anywhere and still come up with tons of tasty information about the GL Diet.

Part 1: Getting Started

Chapter 1 homes in on why eating the low-GL way makes so much sense, and why GL is here to stay. If you want to take a whistle-stop tour through the last few decades of the low-carb diet world and find out how science has led us to understand that GL is both an effective and healthy way to control weight, head to Chapter 2. Chapter 3 gets down to business with your start-up guide, suggested eating plans, and ways to fit in all the other elements of a healthy diet.

Part II: Shopping and Eating Out

In Chapter 4 you get the lowdown on getting in and out of the supermarket with everything you need and nothing you don't, simply buying fantastically healthy food to keep you in the driving seat where your weight is concerned. You can also find the best choices when eating on the run or grabbing a quick lunchtime bite. Chapter 5 takes you on a round the world trip of eating out GL-style, from Indian to Mexican food.

Part III: Morning to Night Recipes

Head to Chapter 6 for breakfast recipes to suit every taste and give you the perfect start to your low-GL day. Chapter 7 has low-GL lunches in a box for the office or out on the run, as well as delicious lunches to have at home. You'll find Chapter 8 full of our favorite dinner recipes; some that you can pop on the table in minutes and others that you can take your time over or dish up for a special occasion. Chapter 9 spills over with delicious desserts, and Chapter 10 has nutrient-packed snacks for those in-between times.

Part IV: Optimising GL

Want to know how to mix high- and low-GL foods to control the overall GL of a meal? Jump to Chapter 11. Chapter 12 explains where GL fits into the other aspects of healthy living, and also looks at getting your head in the right place to make positive changes to your lifestyle. Skip to Chapter 13 for the health benefits of the GL Diet, so even if you don't want to lose weight, you can really see how your health can benefit from eating the low-GL way.

Part V: The Part of Tens

You can't have a *For Dummies* book without The Part of Tens! This part gives you ten positive health benefits of eating low GL, plus ten great sources of help, support, and further information along with the Web address to get you there quickly. You can also find ten super-easy food swaps to get you around any high-GL food dilemma.

Icons Used in This Book

Icons are a handy *For Dummies* way to catch your attention as you slide your eyes down the page. The icons come in several varieties, each with its own special meaning:

This little guy looks smart because he marks the place where you find explanations of the terms used by GL experts.

This masked marvel cuts through the diet myths to let you know the truth.

Check out these snippets of useful information that you want to bear in mind.

This icon alerts you to clear, concise explanations of technical terms and processes – details that are interesting but not necessarily critical to your understanding of a topic. In other words, skip them if you want, but try a few first.

Bull's-eye! This highlights time- and stress-saving information that you can use to improve your low-GL lifestyle.

The bomb alerts you to pitfalls where you need to take extra care.

Where to Go from Here

Ah, here's the best part. You don't have to read a *For Dummies* book from cover to cover. In fact, you can dive right in anywhere and still make sense of what you're reading because we make sure that each chapter delivers a complete message.

If you want to know the best low-GL choices in your local Italian place, go right to Chapter 5. If you've always been fascinated by eating for health, your choice is Chapter 13. Want to cook a low-GL dinner tonight? Pick your favourite recipe from

Chapter 8. You can use the Table of Contents to find broad categories of information or the Index to look up more specific things.

If you're not sure where you want to go, you may want to start with Part I. The chapters here give you all the basic information that you need to understand the GL Diet and points to places where you can find more detailed information.

Part I
Getting Started

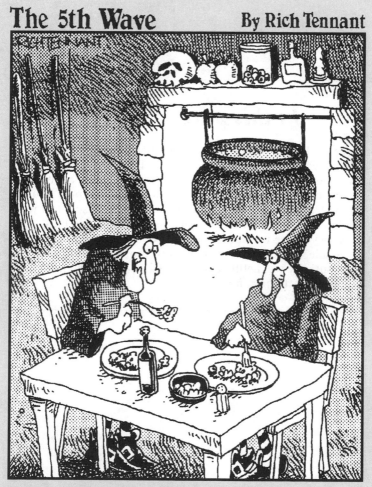

The 5th Wave By Rich Tennant

"Oooo, what's in here? Is that sun-dried eye of newt? How gourmet!"

In this part . . .

*P*art I gives you everything you need to start your low-glycaemic load eating plan. You'll find an overview of the science behind GL and why we think it's such an important tool for a healthy, happy way of eating that puts you in control of your weight and well-being. You'll see how we added all the other elements of a healthy diet and lifestyle to give you the very best and most complete information available. If you want to satisfy your inquiring mind and find out why we dietitians like the GL approach so much, then this is the part for you.

Chapter 1

Introducing GL: Healthy Eating in the Real World

. . . .

In This Chapter

▶ Discovering a healthy eating plan that makes scientific sense

▶ Understanding the key principles of easy GL eating

▶ Putting the pieces into practice

▶ Embracing the GL lifestyle for good health – for keeps

▶ Hearing from the professionals

. . . .

*T*he diet industry is worth millions because people are con-tinually searching for that elusive perfect diet. Diet fads come and go; some diets are effective and some are downright dangerous. Industrialised countries face an obesity epidemic with huge implications in terms of individual suffering and medical costs. Therefore, people turn in hope to the latest eating trends fuelling the quest for the perfect diet – diets that seem to become more and more extreme.

Working with patients, training the dietitians of the future, and sifting through the mountain of scientific evidence surround-ing different dietary theories means that we can see the prob-lem of finding an effective diet from many different angles.

We work with people who need help improving their diet and lifestyle, and we have access to the evolving science along with the skills to translate new findings into real-life strategies and real foods. As registered dietitians, we're at the frontline in the battle to find a diet that's satisfying, good for you, and promotes a healthy weight. We have great news for you – we've found it!

In this chapter we introduce you to the *Glycaemic Load Diet* (GL Diet), the most significant breakthrough in nutritional science by far. The GL Diet is balanced and provides all the nutrition you need to be healthy. We share with you why the easy-to-follow low-GL way of eating can give you more energy, reduce your risk of disease, stamp out your food cravings, and enable you to maintain a healthy weight.

Weight-loss diets often forget about the complete nutritional package you need to achieve not only a healthy weight but a healthy body, too. The GL Diet is sustainable for life – that means it's both safe and nutritionally complete.

Easy to Choose, Easy to Use

The GL Diet is based on eating certain carbohydrates, as part of a healthy diet, that slowly release energy keeping you going for longer, rather than storing the fuel away as fat. (Head to Chapter 2 for more of the science behind the eating plan.)

One of the best things about the GL-way of eating is the flexibility that you have with food. Whether or not you're trying to lose weight, you won't feel at all as if you're on a restrictive diet. Think of the GL Diet as an eating plan, rather than a diet – much nicer!

The two most important factors for healthy eating are:

- ✔ **Enjoy your food:** Eating is a pleasant aspect of your life. The GL Diet doesn't ban any foods nor make other foods obligatory. Enjoying your food the GL-way means getting a better balance of foods in your diet in order to be healthy and to minimise the risk of disease.

- ✔ **Eat a variety of foods:** The greater the variety of foods you eat, the more essential nutrients your diet will contain, especially the necessary vitamins and minerals.

These two concepts are the very pinnacle on which to base a healthy, happy, balanced diet. The idea of avoiding any food forever fills us both with horror. As well as being registered dietitians, we're also both real foodies. We love to cook and we love to eat – and that's why we love GL.

Putting GL into Practice

We want to make sure that you have everything you need to start the GL Diet today – hassle-free. We spent hours searching the supermarket aisles for GL-friendly foods; we picked our way through loads of restaurant menus to help you eat out in GL-style (the hard life of a *For Dummies* author); and we hit the kitchen to develop a range of recipes so that you can eat low GL all the way.

Low-GL food guides

You'll find lots of information about choosing food for your low-GL eating plan in Chapters 11, 12, and 16. Here are some at-a-glance guidelines:

- **Meat, fish, and poultry:** Choose a good mixture of protein foods including lean meats, skinless poultry, and a mix of white and oily fish.

- **Fruit and vegetables:** Pretty much all fruit and veg are great on a low-GL diet (take a look at the Cheat Sheet). Aim to eat a rainbow of different colours to get the best mix of vitamins and minerals.

- **Fats:** Replace saturated fat (such as butter and lard) with polyunsaturated (such as corn oil) and monounsaturated fats (such as olive oil).

- **Nuts and seeds:** All nuts and seeds are good for you and for your low-GL plan in moderate quantities.

- **Grains:** Go for the wholegrains such as oats, pearl barley, rye, and bulgur wheat.

- **Pasta, rice, and potatoes:** Choose small amounts of pasta and don't overcook it. Mix rice with lentils or beans to lower the GL, and choose small new potatoes or sweet potatoes over large white potatoes.

- **Breads:** Pick the grainiest bread possible, because bread with seeds and nuts is lower GL than white or wholemeal bread.

Shopping low-GL style

Some diets force you to buy and eat a whole new range of foods you'd never normally touch. In fact, many people gave up on their diets because they simply don't like the food they have to eat.

The good news is that the GL Diet doesn't come with a lot of rigid rules or foods that are banned.

Successful shopping low-GL style relies on some very simple principles:

- ✔ Be prepared – always shop with a list based on the foods you need for the next few days
- ✔ Never shop when you're hungry
- ✔ Don't be tempted by special offers on food that you don't need. If you don't need it, don't buy it!

Read Chapter 4 for more about getting in and out of the supermarket in one healthy, happy piece.

The Cheat Sheet at the front of this book gives you a handy guide to the best low-GL options for starchy staples and seasonal fruits and veggies. Be sure to check it out, or better yet, tear it out and keep it with you.

Eating out, eating well

Eating out is the perfect way to catch up with friends – and all the gossip! The last thing you want when you hope to have a good time is to deprive yourself by nibbling on a lettuce leaf – simply because you're not sure of your low-GL options.

Take these golden nuggets to heart to help you stay on track no matter where you're dining:

- ✔ When you take your seat, ask for some water. A drink of water wards off the hunger pangs.
- ✔ Avoid grazing on the bread basket, which is probably full of high-GL breads.

> ✔ Don't starve all day as an allowance for a blow-out at dinnertime.
>
> ✔ Ask for exactly what you want; you're the customer after all. Sauce on the side instead of poured over your dinner? Fruit or cheese for dessert? Just a small portion of pasta? You call the shots!

When preparing to write this book, we ate out in Chinese, Indian, Mexican, and fast-food restaurants so that we could give you the latest low-GL menu choices available. Chapter 5 is your whistle-stop tour of what's GL-hot and what's not in your favourite restaurants. All that research was tough, but hey, someone had to do it.

Recipes for success

Knowing the foods that are low-GL is useful, but you also need to have recipes for preparing low-GL foods. Check out Part III, where you find heaps of low-GL recipes that will make your mouth water.

We combine our dietitians' hats and our chefs' hats to create a wide range of great low-GL dishes to cook at home. We use simple, everyday ingredients, and you don't need to be a cordon bleu chef to make any of them – the recipes are quick, nutritious, easy to make, and delicious. By simply substituting one ingredient for another – such as using fructose instead of sugar – you can really lower the GL of some of your favourite recipes. We include plenty of fruit and vegetables in our recipes to help you towards achieving your five portions a day, and we include dairy foods to help keep your bones healthy.

Our recipes include a good mix of protein foods from both animal and vegetable sources, so we cater to you vegetarians, as well. We pull no punches with salt and sugar – if our recipe doesn't need them, you won't find them.

In Chapter 3 we give you everything you need to start your new GL healthy eating plan, and we make the process as simple and straightforward as possible. After a few weeks of feeling the benefits of eating low-GL you won't need our help any more – you can cruise the supermarket aisles with confidence, dine out in real GL-style, and know how to adapt certain foods to make them more GL friendly.

Completing the Healthy Lifestyle Picture

The food you eat is only part of the story of controlling your weight and staying healthy. We love the GL Diet, but to make your healthy lifestyle complete you need to ensure that physical activity is an integral part of your life. If you're overweight, losing just 5 per cent of your body weight has significant health benefits. Turn to Chapter 12 for the lowdown on getting active the fun and easy way.

Another part of the healthy lifestyle jigsaw is enjoying a good relationship with food. Perhaps developing the mindset to make a positive change to your lifestyle is one of the biggest hurdles that you need to overcome. In Chapter 12, we look at the emotional aspect of eating and give you some smart moves on how to keep your head in the right place and tips on handling guilt, which can put you on the path to getting your body in good shape, and keeping it that way.

Sometimes, when you decide to get your act together your mind can jump in and put a spanner in the works by finding reasons why not to do the right thing. You know what happens if you do what you've always done – that's right, you get what you've always got!

A healthy body comes from a healthy lifestyle. No magic wand or quick fix exists, but small changes really do count.

Listening to the Pros

Health professionals advise their patients about how to include the principles of low-glycaemic eating to help control weight and diabetes. Major food retailers recognise the validity of the low-glycaemic message with food labelling and advice to customers.

The Harvard School of Public Health is lobbying the United States Department of Agriculture (USDA) to change the current recommended Food Pyramid model to one based on low-glycaemic foods. (For the revised food pyramid, see the

Harvard School of Public Health Web site at `www.hsph.harvard.edu/nutritionsource/pyramids.html`.) The World Health Organisation (WHO) and Food and Agriculture Organization of the United Nations (FAO) recommend that people in industrialised countries base their diets on low-glycaemic foods in order to prevent coronary heart disease, diabetes, and obesity.

The GL Diet is not simply a 'here today, gone tomorrow' fad. It's a diet that's here to stay. The GL Diet takes a difficult, scientific concept and relates the idea to our everyday lives, for our overall improved health.

Chapter 2

Checking Out the Science behind GL

Carbohydrates or carbs for short – bread, rice, potatoes, pasta, and cereals, as well as sugars, confectionary, and, to some degree, alcohol – certainly have their share of the headlines. Once considered the mainstay of any healthy diet, carbs became public enemy number one overnight and a plethora of carb-cautious, low-carb, and no-carb diet books hit the shelves.

In this chapter we take a brief look at the carbohydrate revolution. We mainly give you the facts behind the low-carb hype. We also give you the science behind the GL Diet, so that you can impress all your friends with your technical knowledge but also – and most importantly – so that you can benefit from knowing the science of how the diet works.

Making the Connection between Carbs and Weight Gain

Carbohydrates are composed of carbon, hydrogen, and oxygen and are sugar compounds mainly made by plants when plants are exposed to light. Carbs fall into two categories:

- ✓ **Simple carbohydrates** are carbohydrates with only one or two units of sugar. Some simple sugars, but by no means all, are digested quickly to provide instant energy. Simple sugars include sucrose (table sugar) and lactose (milk sugar).

- ✓ **Complex carbohydrates,** also known as *polysaccharides*, have more than two units of sugar linked together. Complex carbs are generally digested more slowly than simple sugars and include starches found in potatoes, breads, pasta, rice, and cereals. Within this group of carbs is a huge variation in the speed at which they're digested.

  - **Dietary fibre** aids digestion because it passes through the system without being used for energy (because human digestion can't break the bonds holding the sugar units together).

Your body runs on *glucose* (also a single unit of sugar). All the digestible carbohydrates you get from food provide either glucose or sugar units that are quickly converted to glucose. The glucose is carried into your cells with the help of *insulin*, a hormone produced in your pancreas.

You store a small amount of carbohydrate energy (called *glycogen*) in your muscles and liver. Glycogen is your instant access power store for when you need immediate bursts of energy. These glycogen storage units have limited space and fill up quickly. When your glycogen stores are full, the only way you can store excess energy is as fat. Too much energy from sugar means more energy storage as fat.

Sugar is a really small, simple molecule that needs little digesting before you quickly absorb it into your bloodstream. Your *blood sugars*, which give you the energy your body needs to function properly, are finely balanced. If your blood sugar levels get too high or too low at any given moment, your body has a contingency plan to deal with the problem. The powerful hormone *insulin* helps keep your blood sugars balanced by mopping up excess sugar. When you eat sugary foods, if you don't need a burst of immediate energy, the excess sugar is stored for later use as fat.

Unstable blood sugars make you much more prone to 'grazing' on high-sugar treats (snacking) between meals. A sharp rise in blood sugar when you snack is followed by a quick fall, and you're left feeling hungry and looking for your next sugar fix. All that sugar means just one thing – you guessed it, more fat storage.

Some carbohydrates, such as bread, rice, and potatoes, have very similar effects on your blood sugars as the simple sugars; such as the white stuff you put in your coffee. Understanding the principle of how carbohydrates affect us was the basis for a diet revolution – the Glycaemic Index, and then the Glycaemic Load.

The Low-down on Low-Carb Diets

During the 1980s and 1990s the world became carb-phobic, and with this fear of carbs, protein became the dieter's best friend.

Low-carb diets work in the short-term, but have unpleasant effects. You can lose weight on a low-carb diet because of a phenomenon called *ketosis* – the breakdown of your body's own protein and some fat to provide glucose for energy. When your liver and muscles have used all their stored glucose for energy, your body starts to melt down its own tissues to keep functioning – sounds gruesome, eh? When you're on a low-carb diet, these empty glucose stores never get a chance to fill up.

Ketosis is hard work for your body and this condition is not the ideal way for your system to function. Although you eat plenty of protein on a low-carb diet, your body still attacks itself to make energy when carbs are lacking in your diet. Those 7 or 8 pounds you're so proud to have lost in just seven days are actually, at best, 1 or 2 pounds of fat, and 5 or 6 pounds of your own lean-muscle tissue, water, and valuable minerals. In fact, one of the main by-products of ketosis is water so most of your weight loss has gone, well, down the toilet!

The rise and fall of the Atkins empire

Dr Robert C. Atkins was one of the first people to put his head above the parapet and say, 'Maybe weight gain isn't just about fat and calories.' Atkins's timing was perfect; just as the world was looking for a new diet revolution, the Atkins Diet appeared and became one of the biggest-selling books ever seen – even out-selling the Bible! Atkins introduced the concept of carbohydrate management, but his message focused on limiting the total amount of carbohydrates you eat (including some fruits and vegetables), while eating unlimited amounts of protein and often high-fat food.

The principle of eating high-fat food opened Atkins to widespread criticism. Medical and nutrition professionals could not accept that strictly limiting an entire food group (carbs) while freely eating foods laden with calories and unhealthy fats was safe, maintainable, or acceptable.

Sadly, Dr Atkins died in April 2003 and in 2005 the Atkins corporation went bankrupt. By then, nutritionists had begun to understand that carbohydrate management was more complex than just cutting out carbs completely.

When you return to eating a more balanced diet including more carbs, your body devours and retains those needed materials and the weight zooms straight back on, quite often to a greater degree than before you started the diet.

As well as putting your body into a state of ketosis, the effects of a high-protein, high-fat diet on your heart and kidneys is of concern. Your kidneys are critical for removing excess protein from the body, and can become overloaded on a high-protein diet, making them less efficient at removing waste products from the blood, which can be fatal. If you consume a diet high in saturated fats from animal products, you may suffer from high cholesterol, which can cause arteries to fur up and put stress on your heart.

The good news is that the low-carb era captured the imagination of nutritionists who could see that they needed to investigate carbohydrates and their digestion more thoroughly.

In doing so, the nutritionists looked at the different rates at which some carbohydrates were broken down to create glucose and the response that this rate of conversion caused in insulin production. The nutritionists named the process of food being absorbed into the bloodstream as glucose, the *glycaemic response.*

Turning to the Glycaemic Index

The *Glycaemic Index (GI)* is a scientific test that measures how long your body takes to convert carbohydrate from the time that you put food into your mouth, to the time that the glucose is stored in your cells. Foods that quickly turn from carbs to glucose (high-GI foods) cause a sharp rise or *spike* in blood sugars and a rapid insulin response. Your blood sugars fall again after the insulin has stored the glucose in your cells, leading to a slump in your energy levels (see Figure 2-1). Foods that slowly convert their carbs into glucose (low- or moderate-GI foods) cause a more gentle production of insulin and provide long-lasting energy.

The nutritionists also found that the carbohydrate foods that turn to glucose in your cells quickly also trigger hunger more quickly, whereas the slow carbs are more satisfying and result in less hunger.

The Glycaemic Index (GI) is an important scientific reference to gauge your body's response to the carbohydrates you consume. Based on the effect that carbs have on your blood sugar, nutritionists classify foods with the Index, and each food is categorised as low-or high-GI. (See the sidebar 'Delving deeper into the science of GI' if you want to know more about the science behind the Glycaemic Index.)

Stable blood sugars are one of the main factors that make a low-glycaemic diet so helpful in weight control, because stable blood sugars and sustained energy are linked to fewer food cravings.

The Glycaemic Index is a great foundation for understanding the Glycaemic Load, but GI has flaws that you need to be aware of.

Delving deeper into the science of GI

The Glycaemic Index was created by comparing the blood sugar levels of volunteers after eating different foods. After an overnight fast, volunteers ate a quantity of food that provided 50 grams of energy-providing carbohydrates. Nutritionists took blood samples from the volunteers at 15- to 30-minute intervals over the next 2 hours to ascertain the volunteer's blood sugar and insulin response to the test food. Nutritionists compared the results with the response caused by consuming 50 grams of pure carbohydrate (usually glucose). Nutritionists then gave each food a number depending on how fast the body absorbed the carbs – the high the number, the faster the absorption. The number is called the food's Glycaemic Index or GI.

The Glycaemic Index has three categories, and all foods fall into any one of the categories:

✔ GI of less than 55 = Low GI

✔ GI of 56–70 = Moderate GI

✔ GI of 71–100 = High GI

Don't panic! You don't have to worry about working out GI or do any other counting in this book – we've done all that work for you.

All those GI values can be downright confusing; we've seen people get mixed up about whether the GI means calories, amounts of sugar, or even fat. Like counting calories, working out the GI of your meal is impractical and boring. The Glycaemic Index tests the amount of food needed to provide the body with 50 grams of useable carbohydrate, which may be much more or much less than you would ever eat in one sitting. Trying to weigh the ingredients of your meal to get the 50 grams of carbohydrate can give a misleading and confusing result.

Using the Glycaemic Load (GL) to help you to eat healthily is much more sensible and much easier. You don't have to count GLs (unless you really want to) – GL deals with the food on your plate rather than using complex weights and references. The food lists, shopping guide, eating-out guide, and of course the recipes in this book save all the confusion and effort. Eat regularly, take some activity every day, follow our eating plan, and you're living the GL life already!

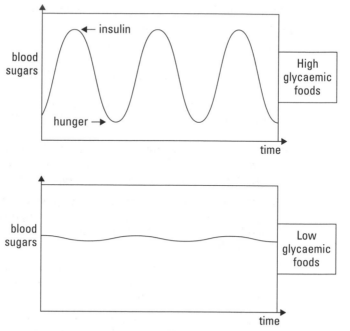

Figure 2-1: A comparison of low- and high-GI food on blood sugar.

Welcome to the Glycaemic Load Story: Real Portions, Real Food

The Glycaemic Load (GL) is derived from a mathematical equation developed by Professor Walter Willet, Chairman of the Department of Nutrition at Harvard Medical School. GL is based on the Glycaemic Index (GI) but also factors in the carb content of an *average portion size*. In other words, GL translates GI into real food portion sizes making the method simpler and more applicable to the way you actually eat. The Glycaemic Load is the final part of the carbohydrate jigsaw.

GL is more effective than GI in a number of ways:

- ✔ GL relates to normal portions of food
- ✔ GL means more food choices
- ✔ GL does not restrict healthy foods

✔ GL means that you don't have to weigh food

✔ GL gives the whole picture of how carbohydrates affect blood sugars

The GL gives you an accurate and sensible picture of what really happens when you eat carbs. Here's how we work it out, but remember, you don't have to worry about any of the maths, or do any of the counting yourself. We've done it all for you.

✔ First take the GI rating of the food. The Web site www. glycaemicindex.com gives you all the latest GI-rated foods and their carbohydrate concentration.

✔ Divide that number by 100. For example, carrots have a high GI of between 75 and 85, depending on how old the carrots are and how long you cook them for (75 divided by 100 = 0.75).

✔ Multiply that number by the actual carbs in an average portion. (100 grams of carrots contains around 7 grams of carbs. 0.75 × 7 = GL of 5.25.)

✔ 100 grams of carrots is a normal portion, but to get 50 grams of those crucial useable carbs from carrots for GI testing you need about 750 grams or 1½ pounds of carrots, which might be normal if you're a donkey, but is probably a bit on the heavy side for likes of us humans.

The GL ratings classification is:

✔ Low GL = 10 or less

✔ Moderate GL = 11–19

✔ High GL = 20 or more

The bottom line when it comes to GL and carrots (and loads of other foods for that matter) is that a normal portion of carrots with a GL of 5.25 is low and means that we can eat carrots with confidence as a good, nutritious, healthy food. Now isn't that a more sensible approach than GI?

Chapter 3

Starting Your Low-GL Plan

. . . .

In This Chapter

▶ Making the change to a low-GL way of eating

▶ Coping with relapse

▶ Getting started with ideas from sample daily meal plans

▶ Combining GL with nutritious eating for optimal health

. . . .

You've made up your mind to give low-GL eating a go – congratulations. You can look forward to feeling more energised, experiencing fewer food cravings, and achieving a healthy, stable weight. You're raring to go, but where do you start? And how does low-GL eating fit together with other aspects of a healthy diet?

In this chapter we help you find the answers to both of these questions. We take you step by step through the process of making the dietary change towards including low-GL foods in your daily life. We provide you with some examples of low-GL alternative eating in our sample meal plans, and show you how a low-GL diet fits simply and easily alongside other recommendations for healthy eating.

Changing Your Diet the Simple and Successful Way

Changing your established behaviour patterns is never easy, and changing what you eat is no exception.

As registered dietitians, we've learnt from experience that you need strategies to help you make and maintain dietary changes. The following list is a summary of your action plan for undertaking this change:

✔ **Establish your goals:** Decide on what you want to change about your diet.

✔ **Plan your actions:** Settle on what you are going to do to achieve your goals.

✔ **Overcome the barriers:** Find out how to get around the things that prevent you from changing your diet.

✔ **Prevent relapse:** Get back on track when you start to waver.

The following sections describe your action plan in more detail, putting you on the path to make eating the low-GL way second nature.

Setting SMART goals

As a first step to changing your current eating plan towards a low-GL diet, you need to decide what changes you want to make and translate these changes into goals that you aim for. Make sure that your goals are *SMART* for maximum effectiveness.

To illustrate what we mean by this term we use goals about fruit and vegetables because they are a vital part of a low-GL way of eating. Make your goals:

✔ **Specific.** Make your goals clear and not too general. Replace 'Eat more healthily' or 'Eat more fruit and vegetables' with 'Eat five portions of fruit and vegetables a day'.

✔ **Meaningful.** Make sure that your individual goals have a beneficial effect on your overall diet. For example, having a goal of drinking a carton of fruit juice a day is specific but isn't very meaningful in terms of the overall health benefit. You need five fruit and vegetable portions a day. Juice of any type only counts once (check out the section 'What's a portion?').

✔ **Acceptable.** You don't have to eat anything you don't like simply because the nutritional content is good for you, or because someone tells you that you ought to eat it. With the low-GL way of eating no food is compulsory and better still, no food is banned. The GL Diet is all about eating normal food, with nothing odd or unpleasant – and no cabbage soup!

✔ **Realistic.** The goals you set for yourself need to stretch you but not so much that you can't achieve them. As a golden rule, avoid setting any goal that begins with the words 'I will never' or 'I will always'. Tell yourself 'I will always have fruit instead of dessert' and you're setting yourself up for failure because you feel as if you're deny-ing yourself. Instead, tell yourself 'I will enjoy a small dessert when I feel I've deserved it and not feel guilty about it'. Be kind to yourself and build some flexibility into your goals. Allow yourself some treats along the way.

✔ **Tailored to you.** We don't know about you, but in our opinion, to have any chance of lasting, a realistic dietary change has to fit properly into your lifestyle, not vice versa. If you don't have time available every day to shop for or prepare fresh fruit and vegetables, an alternative goal is to ensure that you stock up once a week on a com-bination of fresh fruit and veg, ready-to-use products, and a selection of frozen and canned fruit and vegetables.

Planning action

Now that you've set your goals, think hard about how you're going to achieve them. For example, to help you achieve the goal of eating five different servings of fruit and vegetables a day, think about fulfilling this target by:

✔ **Changing the *quantity* of the food, or types of food you eat.** You can increase the amount of fruit and veg you eat at a meal. If you usually have one vegetable with your evening meal, add another. If you usually have one piece of fruit in your lunch box, try two. This simple step increases your fruit and veg quota with very little effort.

If you love high-GL foods, such as white varieties of bread, pasta, and rice, eat them in smaller portions or simply less often.

✔ **Changing the *frequency* of eating certain foods.** You can increase how often you eat fruit and vegetables. If you don't have fruit or vegetables at every meal, try doing so for a few days and see how easy making this change can be. Have a glass of juice with breakfast, or add some sliced fruit to your cereal. Pop a couple of tomatoes into your lunch box or make sure that you serve a salad with pasta at dinner. Similarly, you can *reduce* the frequency of eating certain foods. If you usually have a chocolate bar every day as a snack, save it for a treat on Fridays. You'll enjoy it all the more.

Keep a food diary for a few days so you can check back to see how you're doing.

✔ **Changing the *types* of foods you eat.** You can change the types of foods you eat within a food group. Don't get stuck using the same fruit and vegetables – try including a wide variety of low-GL choices and you're more likely to reach the goal of eating five portions a day.

Replace high-GL refined white bread, pasta, and rice with low-GL wholegrain varieties such as seeded breads, brown basmati rice, bulgur wheat, or couscous. If you love potatoes, try new potatoes or sweet potatoes instead (or have a smaller portion).

See the Appendix for a list of low-GL fruit and vegetables and Chapter 16 for savvy food swaps.

Pulses and beans are wonderful low-GL foods, and can be considered a vegetable towards part of your five-a-day, though multiple portions can only count once (see the section 'What counts towards my five a day?').

Small changes *do* count. Making several small improvements to your diet over time has an amazing ripple effect as the benefits of your efforts accrue and really start to make a difference to your health.

Overcoming Barriers to Change

Changing your diet isn't just about knowing what you should and shouldn't eat – the healthy choice also has to be an easy choice, otherwise your eating plan becomes difficult to sustain.

Think carefully to identify the barriers that may stop you from changing your diet and maintaining healthy eating in the long term.

Your barriers and their possible solutions may include:

- ✔ **Your lack of time to shop.** If you have difficultly carrying home all the fruit and vegetables your family needs, and your local corner shop doesn't carry much stock, you can set up a supermarket home-delivery service (check out the Web sites of the major supermarkets). Even better, you can register for a local organic fruit and vegetable box scheme, which delivers seasonal produce weekly to your door. Check out `www.alotoforganics.co.uk/cats/organic-vegetables.php` for a list of vegetable delivery services.

- ✔ **Your lack of time to cook.** If you're pushed for time during the week, set aside some time to cook in bulk and then freeze the meals. You can simply reheat the meals as you need them. Stock up on convenience items such as quick-cook grains, fresh pasta and sauces, chunky vegetable soups, and canned pulses. If you're really rushed, you can improve the GL of a ready meal or shop-bought pizza by serving with an extra portion of canned, frozen, or fresh vegetables, or a bag of salad.

- ✔ **Your lack of cooking skills.** Eating well doesn't necessarily involve following complex recipes. We include loads of quick and easy recipes in Part III. Keep a look-out for other quick, low-GL recipes in magazines or on the Internet (check out the Web sites we suggest in Chapter 15). If you use good quality fresh ingredients you can often put together a delicious dish with minimal preparation.

- ✔ **Your lack of money to spend on fresh ingredients.** Buying fruit and vegetables and even meat and fish in season is always cheaper. Look out for special offers and bulk buys that you can freeze or store. Farmer's markets and food co-ops are great places to shop economically. If you have green fingers you can even try growing your own in the garden or on an allotment. (Gardening is great exercise too!)

- ✔ **Your likes and dislikes.** Why not experiment and try a new food once a week? Try a new vegetable as an accompaniment or in a soup; a new pulse or bean in a salad; or one of the more unusual low-GL grains instead of pota-toes or bread. Not every food will be a success but over time you can build up a whole new range of low-GL addi-tions to your diet.

Take the time to explore your own barriers and the options available to you. Lateral thinking and planning can really help you overcome your obstacles to change.

Seeking support

You're more likely to succeed with your dietary change, as with any other behavioural change, if you get support from friends and family. A low-GL way of eating is naturally healthy and suitable for anyone, so ask the rest of your household or workplace to get on board with the GL Diet.

If you have a colleague at work who's also a low-GL convert, try taking turns to make a packed lunch for the pair of you.

Dealing with relapse

For most people, a normal part of dietary change is to experi-ence an occasional relapse back into old, unhealthy habits, whether for a meal, a day, or a whole week of Christmas par-ties. The important thing is to accept that your diet won't always be perfect and put the relapse behind you.

Try to work out what may trigger a relapse, to help prevent you going through the whole cycle again. Were you feeling stressed after a bad day at work or bored at home with noth-ing to do? After you pinpoint your triggers to unhealthy eating habits you can take steps to avoid the triggers in the future. Plan how else you can deal with stress or boredom. Eat regular meals and low-GL snacks so that you avoid getting so hungry that you give in to food cravings. If you know that a particular food shop always tempts you in, avoid walking past it.

Experiencing relapse is a normal part of dietary change, so forgive yourself, and get back on track as soon as you can. Head to Chapter 12 for more on the emotional aspect of food.

Something smells fishy . . .

Fish of all sorts can play a fantastic role in a low-GL diet, but oily fish are particularly rich in nutritious fatty acids. Many people say they'd love to eat more oily fish but that they can't be bothered fiddling with the bones or hate the lingering smell of cooking.

Canned and smoked fish, such as mackerel, salmon, and sardines, are already cooked and are very versatile in recipes. A good fishmonger can fillet any fresh fish you buy and even provide you with recipe cards.

A Day in the Life of Low-GL: Sample Meal Plans

The preceding sections show you how to set and stick to goals. This section shows you how a few minor changes to your daily diet can make a huge difference to your health, wellbeing, and weight. Are you ready to leap straight into a low-GL lifestyle? The following sample daily eating plans illustrate how simple actions can help you instantly lower the GL of your diet.

Case study one

Jane is a 30-year-old mother of two young children. Breakfast is a rushed meal prior to getting the kids off to school. Lunch is usually a snack at home. Jane nibbles the kids' snacks or a couple of high-GL rice cakes during teatime with the kids. Dinner is a cooked meal including a vegetable, accompanied by a bottle of wine, which she shares with her husband.

Take a look at Table 3-1 to understand how adjusting the quantity, reducing the frequency, and changing the types of food she eats during the day (see the section 'Planning action') can improve Jane's diet.

Table 3-1	Jane's Pre-GL and Post-GL Diet	
Meal	*High GL*	*Low GL*
Breakfast	Cornflakes with raisins and semi-skimmed milk	All bran with dried apricots or berries and semi-skimmed milk
Lunch	Spaghetti hoops on two slices white toast Tinned rice pudding with jam	Large portion of baked beans on one slice soy and linseed toast Fruit yoghurt mixed with nuts and toasted oats
Dinner	Roast chicken, large jacket potato, and peas. Canned peaches in syrup with condensed milk. Half a bottle of sweet white wine	Roast chicken, medium-sized baked sweet potato, peas, carrots, and broccoli. Fresh fruit salad with reduced-fat single cream 1–2 glasses dry white wine
Snacks	Rice cakes, Mars bar, potato crisps	Rye crisp breads with reduced-fat soft cheese spread, cashew nuts, dried apple rings, fresh fruit

Case study two

Tony is a 55-year-old office worker. Tony likes a good breakfast before work but usually just grabs a sandwich at his desk for lunch. Dinner is a takeaway or sit-down meal at a local Indian restaurant, at least a couple of times a week.

A few simple changes, as outlined in Table 3-2, can really improve Tony's diet.

Table 3-2	Tony's Pre-GL and Post-GL Diet	
Meal	*High GL*	*Low GL*
Breakfast	Cocopops with milk Croissants with jam	Porridge with milk and 1 teaspoon fructose Multigrain bread with grilled tomatoes and mushrooms

Meal	High GL	Low GL
Lunch	Large cheese baguette Tortilla chips Can of fizzy drink	Open sandwich of cheese on sourdough bread with a side salad Unsalted peanuts and an apple Can of diet drink or flavoured water
Dinner	Lamb madras, large portion white rice, naan bread, poppadoms, and mango chutney	Lamb and lentil curry, side dish of spinach (saag) with cucumber raita and a small chappati
Snacks	Hot chocolate, coffee, biscuits, pretzels	Tea, coffee, fresh fruit, home made soup, oatcakes with hummus or peanut butter, plain popcorn

Write down your own typical daily eating plan, or list what you had to eat yesterday. Use this list as a starting point to pinpoint simple changes to lower the GL of your diet. Chapter 16 has some more GL savvy food swaps or turn to the Appendix for more low-GL food ideas.

Finding Balance: How the GL Diet Fits into Healthy Eating

As registered dietitians, any eating plan we follow, or recommend to anyone else, must be varied enough to avoid the risk of dietary deficiency and balanced enough to prevent diet-related illness, such as heart disease and cancer. The low-GL way of eating consists of wonderful variety of healthy foods. You don't need to buy any special 'low carb' foods, you don't need to pop any pills, and you don't need to take any nutritional supplements.

If you *only* take into account the GL aspect of your diet, you can find yourself eating meals that are low in refined carbohydrate, wholegrains, and cereal fibre, and high in saturated fat. We show you how to avoid this trap with our favourite recipes and practical eating out and shopping guides in Chapters 4 and 5. However, this section acts as a checklist for helping you follow a balanced diet alongside the principles of low GL eating. We also answer some of the most commonly asked questions about healthy eating.

Facing the fats

Everyone needs a certain amount of fat in their diet to provide essential fatty acids and absorb fat-soluble vitamins, and to make food tasty and palatable. Fats come in two main types: saturated and unsaturated.

- **Saturated fats** generally come from animal sources with two exceptions, coconut and palm oil. Saturated fats are usually solid at room temperature. Research shows that saturated fat raises blood cholesterol and so increases the risk of heart disease, and most people get far too much in their diet. Reducing your intake of butter, cream, full-fat dairy products, cakes, biscuits, and pastry helps restrict saturated fat intake. Cutting down on fatty meats and meat products and replacing them with lean cuts or alternatives such as poultry, game, fish, soya, Quorn (a meat substitute made from mushroom-like protein), nuts and pulses also lowers your saturated fat intake.

- **Unsaturated fats** are commonly derived from plant foods and fish and are in liquid form as oils. Unsaturated fats can help lower blood cholesterol and so protect against heart disease. They come in two main types: *polyunsaturated oils* from sunflower, corn, and soya oils, as well as from seeds, nuts, and fish; and *monounsaturated fats*, found in rapeseed and olive oil, some nuts, and avocados. On a low GL diet, choose unsaturated oils and spreads for cooking and salad dressings.

Recently, scientists have discovered the effects of another group of fats – the *trans fats*. Trans fats are unsaturated fats that have been processed to make them more solid so they can be used more easily in manufactured foods, such as hard margarines, some baked foods, and takeaways. Trans fats also raise blood cholesterol so restricting your intake of trans fat is sensible for your health.

A special kind of fat – omega-3

The particular type of polyunsaturated fat found in fish, known as *omega-3,* can help lower your blood pressure, reduce blood clotting, and help your heart beat in a normal rhythm, all of which help reduce the occurrence of heart attacks, especially in people at high risk such as people with high blood pressure or high cholesterol levels.

Recent evidence also suggests that a deficiency in omega-3 may play a role in the occurrence of mental health problems such as depression, dementia (including Alzheimer's disease), and even learning and behaviour problems in some children.

What is an oily fish and how much should I eat?

A variety of low-GL oily fish all provide omega 3, whether canned, frozen, fresh, or smoked, including:

- ✔ Anchovies
- ✔ Herring
- ✔ Kippers
- ✔ Mackerel
- ✔ Pilchards
- ✔ Salmon
- ✔ Sardines
- ✔ Trout
- ✔ Tuna

Fresh or frozen tuna counts as oily, but canned tuna is not very rich in omega-3.

For clear-cut health benefits, aim to eat a portion of oily fish at least once a week, or more if you're at risk of heart disease. A portion is about 140 grams or 1 small can.

What if I don't eat fish?

Vegetarians can get omega-3 from omega-3 enriched eggs or spreads (check the label). Organic milk is also a relatively good source of omega-3. Oils and seeds such as flaxseeds, linseeds, rapeseed, and some nuts including peanuts, pecans, almonds, and walnuts as well as green leafy vegetables all contain omega-3, although at much lower levels.

The safety of oily fish

Some people worry about possible environmental pollutants in oily fish but recent studies show that the health benefits of eating oily fish outweigh the risks. However, children under 16, and girls and women who are pregnant, breastfeeding, or may become pregnant should avoid eating long-lived fish such as shark, swordfish, and marlin because these fish tend to have higher environmental pollutants such as mercury in their flesh. Women who plan to get pregnant should eat no more than two portions of oily fish a week. This advice also applies to women who are pregnant or breastfeeding. Other women, boys, and men can eat up to four portions per week. For more information see www.food.gov.uk.

If you simply don't enjoy eating fish, try taking omega-3 capsules made from fish-body oil (not the same as cod-liver oil). Aim for around 0.5–1 gram of omega-3 fat per day. Stick to the recommended dose shown on the label. Certain brands are especially formulated for children.

Fitting in the fruit and vegetables

A good intake of fruit and vegetables is central to a low-GL eating plan. As well as being low GL, fruit and vegetables contain a whole cocktail of *phytochemicals* or beneficial nutrients that protect against heart disease and cancer. Studies clearly show the health benefits that can be gained from eating at least five different portions of fruit and vegetables a day.

What counts towards my five a day?

All types of fresh, frozen, tinned, and dried fruit and vegetables can contribute towards your five a day quota. However, fruit juice, dried fruit, and pulses only count once each day because they contain fewer of the protective nutrients. Five glasses of orange juice won't cut it!

Potatoes don't count towards one of your five portions. Potatoes are classed as a starchy carbohydrate instead, along with bread and other cereals. Potatoes, other than baby new potatoes, are also high-GL. All other vegetables are low in GL.

To get the best mix of phytochemicals, eat a variety of colours and create a rainbow of fruit and veg in your diet.

What's a portion?

The following examples show you what counts as one portion:

- 2–3 small fruits, such as kiwis, satsumas, plums, figs, or apricots

- 1 medium fruit, such as an orange, pear, nectarine, banana, or apple

- 1 slice of larger fruit, such as pineapple, melon, or papaya

- 1 handful of berries, such as strawberries, cherries, or grapes

- 3 tablespoons of cooked or tinned fruit

- 1 tablespoon of dried fruit, such as apricots

- A glass (150 millilitres) of 100 per cent fruit juice

- 3 tablespoons of cooked beans or pulses

- 3 heaped tablespoons of cooked vegetables

- 1 small bowl of salad

- Half an avocado or grapefruit

Encourage children to eat at least five different fruits and vegetables each day, but in smaller portion sizes – around a handful.

Can I take a dietary supplement instead?

Unfortunately, we do not recommend taking dietary supplements as a substitute to eating a healthy balanced diet. Pills containing isolated vitamins or minerals do not have the same benefits as actually eating the fruits and vegetables themselves.

Daily dairy

Most dairy foods are low-GL but they can also be high in saturated fat. The best dairy choices are the reduced-fat varieties, such as semi-skimmed milk, low-fat yoghurt, and lower fat cheeses. Low-fat dairy products are just as high in nutrients, such as calcium, as the full-fat varieties.

Dairy foods are the primary source of calcium, providing you with the richest and best-absorbed form of this vital element in your diet. You need an adequate quantity of calcium to maintain strong bones and help prevent osteoporosis or brittle bones in later life. Recent studies show that dairy foods also play a role in helping to lower blood pressure and possibly even help to control body weight.

How much dairy do I need?

Aim for 2–3 servings per day of lower fat varieties of milk, cheese, or yoghurt. A serving is:

- ✔ 1 carton (150 grams / 5 ounces) natural or low-fat Greek-style yoghurt

- ✔ ⅓ pint skimmed or semi-skimmed milk

- ✔ 1 ounce (30 grams) cheese (lower fat types include: feta, mozzarella, ricotta, Brie, Camembert, Gouda, Edam, soft goat's cheese, and reduced-fat hard cheese)

Useful amounts of calcium can also come from cottage or curd cheese, quark (a soft cheese), fromage frais, and low-fat soft cheese and cheese spreads.

What if I don't eat dairy foods?

You can find limited amounts of calcium in tinned bony fish, such as sardines or pilchards, in a variety of nuts, in sesame seeds, green leafy vegetables, dried fruit such as figs, and tap water (if you live in a hard-water area). Higher calcium alternatives include calcium-enriched soya products such as milk, cheese, and yoghurts, soy-bean curd (tofu), calcium-fortified water, or even a daily calcium supplement.

Don't forget fibre

Fibre is a type of carbohydrate. Two types of fibre keep your body healthy:

- ✔ **Soluble fibre** helps to lower cholesterol levels, control blood-sugar levels, and promotes healthy gut bacteria. A low-GL diet is naturally high in soluble fibre found in fruit, vegetables, pulses, oats, and oat bran.

✔ **Insoluble fibre** helps keep the bowel healthy, protecting against bowel cancer and preventing constipation. Whenever possible, ensure that you choose unrefined wholegrain versions of starchy foods such as bread, pasta, rice, or other cereal products. Low GL providers of insoluble fibre include rye or mixed wholegrain or seeded bread, brown basmati or wild rice, wholewheat pasta, and other wholegrains, such as pearl barley, bulgur wheat, and quinoa.

Water, water everywhere

Water carries nutrients around your body, helps you get rid of waste products (via urine), and controls your body temperature (through sweat). Ideally, you need to drink 6–8 glasses or cups of fluid a day; more if the weather's very hot or if you're very active.

The good news is that any fluid, not just water, can contribute towards your total fluid intake. Low GL drinks include milk, coffee, tea, sugar-free squash, low calorie fizzy drinks, and diluted fruit juices. But not all liquids are equally rehydrating. Very strong coffee and the alcohol in beer, wine, and spirits, act as *diuretics*, chemicals that make you urinate more.

A word about salt

Most people eat too much salt in their diet – around 9 grams (one and a half teaspoons) per day. High salt intake may be associated with high blood pressure, so try to keep your intake below 6 grams (1 teaspoon) of salt per day on your low-GL plan. Salt is a chemical compound called *sodium chloride*. All forms of salt, including sea and rock salt, are sodium chloride.

Around three quarters of the salt you eat is hidden in processed foods including cereal products, sauces, ready meals, and takeaways. To help reduce your total intake, check the label for lower salt varieties when buying these foods as part of your low GL diet.

To assess the salt content of a food from the label, simply multiply the sodium by 2.5. So a food product labelled as containing 0.5 grams of sodium has 1.25 grams of salt.

Take a look at the recipes in this book, and you'll see that we use no added salt. We also give you the sodium content in the nutritional analysis of each recipe.

You can cut down on adding salt to your food during cooking and while at the table by using any type of fresh or dried herbs and spices, including black pepper, instead. For dishes that require salt, you can use a salt substitute made from potassium chloride, commonly available in supermarkets.

Part II
Shopping and Eating Out

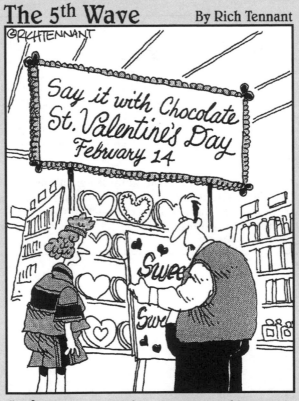

The 5th Wave   By Rich Tennant

Say it with Chocolate
St. Valentine's Day
February 14

"Of course you're better off eating
fish and vegetables, but for St.
Valentine's Day, we've never been very
successful with, 'Say it with trout'."

In this part . . .

Any new eating plan must be easy to follow and fit into your lifestyle if you're going to stick with it. The GL Diet ticks both of those boxes. Part II gives you clear information so that you can shop for low-GL food with confidence. That means that you can buy food you actually want to eat!

In Part II you also take a look at suitable selections for low-GL fast food and drink, as well as exploring the menu options for more leisurely dining out – whatever your favourite type of restaurant is.

Chapter 4

Cruising with Confidence: Low-GL Shopping and Eating on the Run

● ●

In This Chapter

▶ Shopping smart for food that fits the low-GL lifestyle

▶ Stocking up on low-GL basics

▶ Figuring out food labels

▶ Grabbing GL-friendly fast food for eating on the run

● ●

*A*ny eating plan worth its salt must fit easily into your lifestyle to be successful. That's why we've taken out the effort of shopping for low-GL ingredients, and put together handy checklists and shopping tips for wherever you go to buy food. This chapter also gives you some ideas on how to build a store cupboard of low-GL ingredients, and hints on how to help make sense of food labels.

After the shopping, we take you on a cruise around the fast food outlets and sandwich bars for low-GL choices to grab when you're out and about.

Going Low-GL in the Supermarket

When you first switch to a low-GL way of eating, selecting the best choices from each aisle or food group won't always be second nature. Our handy checklists help you build up your own shopping list, and give you ideas for buying a wide variety of ingredients.

Stick to your shopping list! A shopping list helps you stay focused and prevents you wandering off all over the shop getting tempted by all those buy-one-get-one-free offers on jam tarts. Remember that buy-one-get-one-free means BOGOF if it's not an offer on low-GL ingredients! Avoid shopping when you're hungry or thirsty, or you may be tempted to buy all sorts of 'quick-fix' snacks.

So, come with us on a virtual tour of the supermarket aisles. The checklists and shopping tips apply whether you shop in a supermarket or online, and you can use them individually if you're lucky enough to have good local shops, such as a greengrocer, delicatessen, fishmonger, and butcher, or even at a street or farmers' market.

Filling up on fruit and vegetables

The fresh fruit and vegetable aisle (or the local greengrocer or street market) is right at the top of your low-GL shopping list. Remember frozen, dried, and canned fruit and vegetables also count towards your required five portions a day (see Chapter 3 for more on why you're recommended to eat five portions of fruit and veg per day).

When you choose your fruit and vegetables, think about filling your trolley with a rainbow: The greater the variety of colours you buy, the greater the mix of antioxidant nutrients you get to help protect against cancer and heart disease.

Buying loose packed or supermarket-own 'value' brand packs (where the fruit and vegetables may be slightly less than perfect in size, shape, or colour but just as nutritious) are often the cheapest. 'Two-for-one' special offers are economic but only if you can get through the contents before the 'use-by-date'. A popular way of buying fresh products is in the form of ready-to-eat packs of fresh fruit, and salad leaves, and ready-to-cook bags of vegetables for stir-frying or microwaving. You pay for convenience but when time is short the ready packs are a fresh, nutritious, low-GL fast food choice.

Seasonal shopping

When you shop for your fruit and vegetables, bear in mind which varieties are in season, and where the food has been grown. Do you really want asparagus and raspberries in December, flown in from some exotic corner of the globe? If you do, you'll end up paying a premium when you can just as easily get your nutrients from seasonal and locally grown varieties at a fraction of the price.

The vitamin value is also better as local products haven't been sprayed with as many chemicals or stored for long periods of time for transportation. Buying locally, whenever possible, helps the environment, too – saving on the pollution caused by long-haul flights. When you do buy foreign fruit and veg, pick the 'fair-trade' varieties.

You can buy your fruit and vegetables from a local food co-op, which buys in bulk and passes the savings on to the individual. You can even have a weekly fruit and vegetable box delivered to your door. You may not have much say as to what's in the box, but you get a good variety, a few pleasant surprises, and it certainly saves you lugging all those shopping bags home. www.alotoforganics.co.uk/cats/organic-vegetables.php gives you a list of vegetable delivery services.

You can choose from a great variety of some of the lower GL fruits and vegetables shown in Tables 4-1 and 4-2.

Table 4-1	Low-GL Fresh Fruit Checklist		
Apples	Fresh figs	Mangos	Peaches
Apricots	Grapes	Melons	Pears
Bananas (the less ripe, the better)	Grapefruits	Nectarines	Pineapples
Berries (all types)	Kiwis	Oranges	Plums
Cherries	Lemons/Limes	Papayas	Satsumas

Most fresh fruit and fruit tinned in natural juice has a low GL. Dried fruit such as raisins, sultanas, dried figs, and dates are fairly high GL – better choices are dried apples and apricots. Unsweetened juices, other than tomato and carrot, have a moderate GL, so drink a small glass daily or dilute the juice with water.

Table 4-2	Low-GL Fresh Vegetable Checklist		
Artichokes	Carrots	Leeks	Pumpkins
Asparagus	Cauliflower	Lettuce	Radishes
Aubergines	Celery	Mange tout	Rocket
Avocados	Courgettes	Mushrooms	Spinach
Bean sprouts	Cucumbers	Okra	Squashes
Broccoli	Endive	Onions	Swedes
Brussels sprouts	Green beans	Peas	Sweetcorn
Cabbage	Kale	Peppers	Tomatoes

Most vegetables have a low GL and you can eat loads of them without a care. Some root vegetables such as parsnips, sweet potatoes, yams, and cassava have a moderate GL but they still make excellent alternatives to other starchy carbohydrates with a high GL such as mashed potatoes, jacket potaotoes, and chips. You can boil, bake, or mash these alternative root vegetables. Follow these useful tips for buying fruit and vegetables:

- Frozen fruit and vegetables can sometimes have a higher vitamin content than fresh products, which can sit on the shelf or are in transit for some time. Useful purchases include frozen spinach, broad beans, peas, and corn. Berries of all varieties freeze well and are very useful in desserts (see Chapter 9).

- Look for canned fruit and vegetables without added sugar or salt. Low-GL canned veggies include artichoke hearts, water chestnuts, spinach, corn, mushrooms, peas, and, of course, tinned tomatoes.

✔ Beans and pulses are key players in the low-GL diet. Dried varieties need soaking and careful cooking. Tinned varieties are pricier but save you time. Reduce the salt by always draining and rinsing tinned beans and pulses. Select pulses from lentils (red, green, brown, or puy), split peas, and chickpeas. Low-GL beans include kidney, butter, cannelloni, haricot, aduki, butter, borlotti, flageo-let, and pinto. And don't forget low-sugar baked beans!

✔ Seeds are powerhouses of nutrients and are low-GL, too. Choose from sunflower, sesame, flax or linseeds, pump-kin, poppy, and melon. Pine nuts are wonderful toasted in savoury dishes.

✔ Nuts are another great part of a low-GL diet. Choose unsalted wherever possible, including almonds, Brazil nuts, chestnuts, hazelnuts, macadamia, pecans, peanuts pistachios, cashews, and walnuts. You can use ground almonds instead of flour in some baked dishes. Sugar-free peanut butter and reduced-fat coconut milk are useful store cupboard ingredients.

Size matters when buying nuts, seeds, dried fruit, and pulses. Be economical and buy in bulk or loose-packed from a local co-op, ethnic, or wholefood shop rather than at the supermarket. If stored correctly, these ingredients keep fresh for some time.

Choosing meat, fish, and alternatives

All unprocessed meat, poultry, fish, and shellfish are naturally low in carbohydrate and so have a low GL. Choose lean cuts without added cereals or breadcrumbs where possible. Visit your fishmonger, butcher, or the in-store fresh meat and fish counter to see what's in season or on special offer. Don't forget to visit the frozen foods section and check out canned varieties of meat and fish, too.

Table 4-3 is your handy checklist for low-GL choices.

Table 4-3 Low-GL Meat, Fish, and Alternatives Checklist

Canned or fresh crab	Fresh, frozen, or smoked fish (white and oily)	Lean red meat
Canned oily fish	Fresh or frozen shellfish	Offal
Canned tuna	Fresh or frozen squid	Quorn
Chicken portions	Game	Soy mince
Chicken or turkey mince and stir fry pieces	High-meat-content, lean sausages	Tofu
Eggs	Lean mince	Whole chicken

Remember the following tips when you buy meat, fish, and vegetarian alternatives:

- ✔ Fresh fish has clear, bright eyes and moist, firm flesh without any strong or unpleasant odour.

- ✔ Oily fish rich in omega-3 fatty acids include salmon, mackerel, trout, sardines, pilchards, fresh tuna, herring, kippers, and anchovies. Fresh, smoked, frozen and canned varieties are all good for you. We also love ready-to-eat seafood selections for use in sandwiches and salads.

- ✔ Avoid choosing shellfish or white fish in high-GL breadcrumbs or batter.

- ✔ A good butcher can trim your cuts of meat or turn your meat into mince for you to ensure leanness.

- ✔ The supermarket deli counter sells whole roast chickens and a good range of lean, cold cooked meats if you're short of time.

- ✔ Eggs are a great source of protein and very versatile. Choose omega-3 enriched eggs if you don't eat fish.

    Research shows that you can safely eat an egg a day unless you're specifically advised otherwise for medical reasons.

- ✔ Low-GL vegetarian alternatives to meat and fish include tofu (soy bean curd), Quorn (mushroom protein), and soy mince.

Opting for milk and dairy foods

Milk and dairy foods, apart from sweetened and condensed milk, are naturally low in GL but can sometimes be high in saturated animal fat (linked to an increased risk of heart disease). Table 4-4 guides you towards the lower fat choices.

Table 4-4	Low-GL Milk and Dairy Foods Checklist	
Fromage frais	Low-fat single cream	Reduced-fat hard and soft cheese, cottage cheese
Long-life milks and cream	Low-fat sour cream	Skimmed or semi-skimmed milk
Low-fat crème fraîche	Olive oil margarines	Soy milk
Low-fat Greek yoghurt	Parmesan cheese	Yoghurt (bio or natural)

When you buy milk and dairy foods remember:

- ✔ Cheese is high in saturated fat but a little chunk of a really good, mature variety goes a long way. Keep to small portions or choose a reduced-fat cheese such as low-fat mozzarella, cheddar, Edam, or feta.

- ✔ Cottage cheese, low-fat soft cheeses, and cheese spreads are great on bread, used as a pasta sauce, or as an ingredient in cooking.

- ✔ Fresh Parmesan cheese added to a pasta dish helps reduce the GL and adds flavour. Keep a block of Parmesan in the fridge to grate when required.

- ✔ Use cream in moderation and look for reduced-fat varieties where possible, which work very well in most recipes.

Buying bread, cereals, and potatoes

Another food group for your trolley is the starchy foods shown in Table 4-5 – bread, cereals, and potatoes. The choices you make from this group affect the GL of your diet more than any other food group, so follow our tips with extra care.

Table 4-5	Low-GL Bread, Cereals, and Potatoes Checklist	
Bran-based cereals	New potatoes	Sweet potatoes
Brown rice	Oatmeal / porridge oats	Wholegrain, rye, and seeded bread
Buckwheat or kasha	Oat bran	Wholegrain porridge
Bulgur/cracked wheat	Oat cakes	Wholemeal pasta
Couscous	Pearl barley	Yams, celeriac

Here are some tips for when you buy bread, cereals, and potatoes:

✔ Low-GL varieties of bread include those made with 100 per cent wholegrain or wholewheat flour, multi-seeded, soya and linseed, sourdough, rye, or pumpernickel.

✔ Choose rice a with a high *amylose* content, such as long grain, wild, and brown basmati rice, rather than short grain or white sticky rice.

Rice contains two types of starch: *amylose* and *amylopectin*. The GL of amylose is lower because the molecules are packed tightly together, making it take longer to digest.

✔ Wholemeal pasta and fettuccine have a lower GL than most other pasta. Cook your pasta until al dente (still firm when bitten). Mix pasta and rice with beans and pulses to reduce the overall GL, and remember to keep your portions small.

✔ For breakfast, choose from wholegrain oats, oat bran, bran-based cereals, or make your own muesli. We give you a lovely recipe for fast muesli in Chapter 6.

✔ Try adding pearl barley to stews and casseroles or mixed with rice and pasta as an alternative.

✔ Potatoes are a high-GL food. Go for small new potatoes or try mashed or baked celeriac, yam, or sweet potatoes, which have a lower GL.

Some stores have an organic or health food aisle where you may find a better range of low-GL grains and cereals than in the main aisles.

Building a Store Cupboard of Low-GL Ingredients

Stock up on the low-GL staples shown in Table 4-6 and creating meals from your store cupboard stock will be a doddle. We're not suggesting that you stock up on all these ingredients in one go, but just buy one or two items each week and your store cupboard supplies can soon grow.

If you see an interesting low-GL recipe that calls for an ingredient you don't have, add it to your shopping list for the next time you buy food.

Follow these tips for building a low-GL store cupboard:

- Make sure that you have a good supply of cooking and salad oils, preferably those high in monounsaturated fats, which are the most heart friendly. Go for olive, rapeseed, and blended vegetable oil. Add to these staples by buying unusual flavoured oils such as lemon and dill, chilli and garlic, or seed or nut oils such as walnut, soya, peanut, or sesame oil.

- Vinegar is a useful addition to your low-GL diet. Adding an acidic ingredient to your meals such as vinegar slows the digestion of starches and lowers the overall GL. Try balsamic, sherry, and wine vinegars or flavoured varieties, such as tarragon or raspberry. Acidic pickles such as capers, gherkins, sugar free pickles, and sauerkraut also helps lower the GL.

- Dried herbs are useful for times when you can't find fresh. Choose from mixed herbs, coriander, thyme, tarragon, sage, rosemary, oregano, and basil.

- Use spices to pep up the flavour in your food. Delicious examples include cardamom pods, chilli, cumin and coriander seeds, turmeric, ginger, garam masala, cinnamon, Chinese 5-spice, nutmeg, and pepper including paprika, cayenne, and black.

As with pulses, nuts, and seeds you can buy dried herbs and spices most cheaply loose-packed from a self-serve health store to save money.

✔ Low-GL sauces include soy, Worcestershire, Tabasco, chilli sauce, hoi sin sauce, Thai fish sauce, horseradish, and salsa. Look for brands without added sugar.

✔ Pastes are useful additions to your store cupboard for using in sauces. Suggestions include: tahini (sesame seed) for hummus, pesto (basil and pine nuts) for pasta or in a vegetable soup, harissa (hot red pepper) in stews, soups, or couscous, Thai and Indian curry pastes, and black or green olive paste (tapenade) in dips, marinades, or as a spread on bread.

✔ *Fructose*, or fruit sugar, has a lower glycaemic effect than *sucrose* (table sugar) and *glucose* (the simple sugar derived from starchy foods). Use fructose when you need something to sweeten a dish. Fructose is much sweeter than sucrose so use less of it. Unlike some of the artificial sweeteners, fructose gives bulk to foods and so works well in baking.

Table 4-6	Low-GL Store Cupboard Checklist		
Capers	Gherkins	Passata	Sugar-free jams
Curry pastes	Harissa	Pesto	Sugar-free pickles
Dried herbs and spices	Mustard	Pure fruit spreads	Sundried tomatoes
Dried mushrooms	Natural vanilla extract	Sauces (such as soy)	Tahini paste
Flavoured vinegars	Olives	Sauerkraut	Tomato puree
Fructose	Olive paste (tapenade)	Stock cubes	Vegetable/olive/ seed oils

Making Sense of Food Labels

Reading a food label can give you lots of really useful information, but only if you know what to look for – otherwise you can find yourself looking at a foreign language. Food labels are particularly useful for helping you make healthy choices within each food group. With some guidance on interpreting the information on labels and a bit of practice, understanding them becomes second nature.

Investigating ingredients

Once upon a time, the only reliable consumer information on a food label was the name of the food inside in the packet. Now, food labels have an ingredients list that tells you the exact content of the product.

Contents are listed in descending order of weight, so the first item listed is also present in the largest quantity. Watch out for so-called 'healthy desserts', which are lower in fat but surprisingly high in sugar. A scan of the ingredients list helps you get wise to this practice and seek out better alternatives.

Noting the nutritional information

A low-GL way of eating is based on lots of natural and minimally processed foods so, generally speaking, you know that much of the food we recommend is nutritionally sound without even looking at a label. However, you may need to use processed or convenience foods from time to time so understanding how to read the nutritional information on labels is useful. Food labels can help you spot foods particularly high in undesirables such as sugar, salt, or saturated fat. More than 80 per cent of UK-produced, pre-packaged foods have nutritional information on the packaging so you have a wealth of data to help you make careful choices – if you know what the data means!

The nutritional panel on packaged foods lists the main nutrients in the food. Energy is listed as calories (kcal) and kilojoules (kJ); and fat, protein, and carbohydrate are listed in grams. Table 4-7 shows a typical nutritional food label.

Nutritional labels are measured in 100-gram or millilitre portions. Labels also often list nutrients per serving.

The sugar detective

Sugar is hidden in literally hundreds of the processed foods you eat. The nearer sugar appears at the start of the ingredients list, the more sugar is contained in the food in relation to other ingredients. You should be able to easily spot hidden sugar in foods then, right? Well, no, not always. Very often, manufacturers add sugar in several different forms so no one type alone actually shows at the top of the ingredients list. Sometimes, these alternative forms of sugar end in the suffix '-ose', which is simply nutrition speak for sugar. Occasionally, sugars are even more difficult to spot. We list the various disguises for sugar to help you become your own sugar detective. If any of the following ingredients are near the top of the list, or several are present in the list together, you can assume that the food is relatively high in sugar:

- Corn syrup
- Dextrose
- Dried glucose syrup
- Glucose
- Glucose syrup
- Hydrolysed starch
- Invert syrup
- Malt
- Maltose
- Molasses
- Sucrose
- Treacle

Table 4-7	Typical Nutrition Information Panel	
Pasta sauce Typical values	*Per 100 g*	*Per ½ pot*
Energy	279 kJ/67 kcal	418 kJ/100 kcal
Protein	3.0 g	4.5 g
Carbohydrate (Of which sugars)	6.0 g (5.4 g)	9.0 g (8.1 g)

Pasta sauce Typical values	Per 100 g	Per ½ pot
Fat	3.4 g	5.1 g
(Of which saturates)	(0.6 g)	(0.9 g)
Fibre	1.4 g	2.1 g
Sodium	0.4 g	0.6 g
(Salt)	(1.0 g)	(1.5 g)

What's a lot and what's not?

You can use the nutritional information on a food label to tell you whether a food has 'a little' or 'a lot' of a particular nutrient. Table 4-8 shows some rules of thumb developed by the UK Government.

Table 4-8	What Counts as 'a Little' or 'a Lot'?	
Nutrient	A Lot	A Little
Sugar	10 g	2 g
Fat	20 g	3 g
Saturated fat	5 g	1 g
Fibre	3 g	0.5 g
Sodium	0.5 g	0.1 g
Salt	1.5 g	0.3 g

Source: Ministry of Agriculture, Fisheries and Food, 1998

When you look at food labels, consider how often and in what amounts you normally eat the food. A food may be high in saturated fat, but if you only eat small amounts of the product occasionally, you don't need to be concerned that you'll put on loads of weight or increase your risk of heart disease.

Use the 'per 100 g' value to see if food contains a little or a lot of saturated fat, sugar, or salt. You can use the 'per 100 g' or 'per portion' value alongside your knowledge of low-GL to compare similar products, such as ready meals, pasta sauces, and so on to see which is lower unfriendly ingredients. We find keeping a copy of Table 4-8 taped inside our shopping bag useful for quick reference when we need to check a food.

Understanding nutritional claims on food labels

Some foods make claims to be a good source of a particular nutrient ('high fibre', for example), or to contain more or less of the nutrient than a standard item ('low in sugar'). These claims are useful signposts for the busy consumer, but what do 'low' and 'high' actually mean?

Manufacturers must stick to certain guidelines to avoid making misleading claims to the customer. The definitions are still being standardised, but the general consensus is summarised in Table 4-9.

Table 4-9	Guidelines for Nutritional Claims per 100 g or 100 ml
Nutritional claim	*Definition*
Low calorie	40 kcal or less (10 kcal for drinks)
Low sugar	5 g or less
Low fat	3 g or less
Low sodium	40 mg or less
Reduced sugar Reduced fat Reduced salt	Contains at least 25 per cent less than standard product
Sugar free	0.2 g or less

Nutritional claim	Definition
Fat free	0.15 g or less
High fibre	6 g per 100 g or more than 6 g in the amount that you can reasonably eat in a day

Looking at logos

The GI (glycaemic index) symbol is commonly used in Australia (spelled glycemic index) on product labels to help identify low-to-medium glycaemic food choices. (Head to Chapter 2 for more on GI.)

Foods awarded the logo are properly tested and must meet the programme's strict nutrition criteria. This helps consumers to pick out the healthier choices within food categories, and gives a balanced and accurate message about GI.

Some major food manufactures and retailers in the United Kingdom are now recognising the validity of the low glycaemic message and labelling their products as 'low or medium GI', often beside a large 'G'. The logos can help you pick out the lower-GI food within a category such as breads, baked goods, and snack foods.

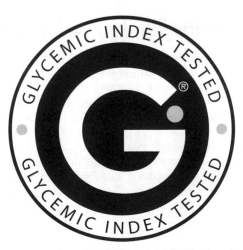

Choosing GL-Friendly Fast Food

Sometimes you don't have time to sit down and enjoy a leisurely meal – you just need a pit stop to grab something quick and easy to fill that gap while on the run. Low-GL choices are still possible in this situation – you just need to know where to look.

Eating on the run

Some fast-food outlets now offer healthy salads. However, skip the high-GL crispy croutons and choose a light dressing.

If you simply can't resist having the occasional burger, try a smaller burger, cheeseburger, grilled chicken sandwich, or even a bean burger. Add some mustard, low-fat mayonnaise, or dill pickles. Discard the top off the burger bun and eat as an open sandwich to reduce the amount of bread. Accompany the burger with a large salad instead of fries.

Go for diet drinks or lower fat milkshakes instead full sugar or full-fat options. Fresh fruit, fruit salad, and yoghurt are good low-GL dessert options. Even the good old-fashioned fish and chip shops offer some lower GL options. Ask for your chicken or fish without the batter. Mushy peas are a great accompaniment, or try a pickled egg or pickled onion.

Smart sandwich-bar selections

Most sandwich bars and coffee shops offer open sandwiches so you can eat less bread, and some shops even provide a 'breadless' sandwich – lean cold meat, tuna, or cheese with salad all wrapped up in lettuce. If bread is the only option, choose the darkest, densest, grainiest bread available.

Look out for pumpernickel, rye, seeded, sourdough, or stone-ground wholegrain bread and ask for thin slices. Ask the staff to use a little light mayonnaise, salad dressing, or mustard instead of butter or margarine. Then fill up your sandwich with some of these low-GL choices:

✔ Lean deli meats, such as roast beef, ham, pastrami, or bacon

✔ Chicken, duck, or turkey

✔ Tuna, prawns, crab, crayfish, or smoked salmon

✔ Low-fat cream cheese or cottage cheese

✔ Chargrilled vegetables

✔ Olives, gherkins

✔ Salad vegetables including spinach, peppers, avocado, onions, rocket, tomatoes, and cucumber

Many sandwich bars also serve soup, which is a satisfying alternative to a sandwich. Select a soup packed with vegetables and pulses, and eat with a small wholegrain roll.

To accompany your meal, choose a packet of popcorn or nuts instead of crisps. Cashews, almonds, or pumpkin or sesame seeds are good GL-friendly choices. A small (20–30 gram) bar of high-cocoa solids dark chocolate can satisfy a sweet tooth, but only indulge yourself now and then.

Sandwich bar dessert options include yoghurt, fruit salad, berries, or fresh fruit. Make sure that you order your coffee without flavoured syrups but for variety try soy milk in your cappuccino or latte. Even better, go for a fruit or herb tea, vegetable juice, a sugar-free smoothie, or bottled water.

Chapter 5

Table for Two? Eating Out GL-Style

. . . .

In This Chapter

▶ Grasping the golden rules for eating out the GL way

▶ Choosing alcoholic drinks wisely

▶ Selecting low-GL dishes from around the world

. . . .

*E*ating out is increasingly popular. On average in the United Kingdom, we lunch or dine out on at least 12 occasions per month, whether in cafes, sandwich bars, fast-food outlets, or restaurants. In the United States, 1 in 5 meals is eaten outside the home – that's an average of 4.2 meals per person per week!

Eating out is one of life's great pleasures. You have the fantastic atmosphere, the great company – and you don't have to do the washing-up (unless you forget your wallet). Last but not least, you have the food. But eating out can be a GL nightmare, with so many refined and carb-heavy choices.

The good news is that you can follow some simple principles to ensure that eating out GL-style is both easy and enjoyable for you. In this chapter, we guide you through a number of useful rules to help you make low-GL choices with confidence. Deprivation isn't on our menu!

Sharing Top Tips for a GL-Friendly Meal Out

Dining out is a treat and you don't want to feel as if you have to follow rigid rules when choosing what to eat. Therefore, we've come up with a few helpful guidelines to help you navigate the menu. Our top tips guarantee you a dining experience that's both tasty and healthy.

Before you order

Before you even browse through the menu, make sure that you've taken the edge off your appetite.

Don't starve yourself all day just because you're going out for a meal in the evening. If you eat nothing all day, you set yourself up to overeat in the evening. Your body naturally starts to wonder where its next meal is coming from, sending your appetite into overdrive and causing you to eat as much as you can when you get the chance.

To prevent yourself from overdoing it, don't arrive at the restaurant with an empty stomach. Have a piece of fruit or a low-fat yogurt before you go out. Say no to the breadsticks and don't delve into the bread basket, which is likely to be brimming with high-GL white bread. If you can't wait for something to eat, ask for a few nuts, olives, or raw vegetable crudités instead.

Drink plenty while you're waiting to order – no, we don't mean wine! You can often mistake the feelings of thirst for those of hunger, and eat too quickly in an attempt to fill up. Ensure that you're really well hydrated before you tuck in to avoid making the mistake of over ordering what you eat. Ask the waiting staff for a jug of ice cold water with lemon, or a bottle of sparkling water if you prefer, and have a couple of glasses while you peruse the menu for delicious low-GL options.

Balancing it out

Look at the menu for smart low-GL choices for the basis for your meal. You can usually find a good range of low-GL options in the meat, poultry, fish, or vegetarian (bean-based) dishes. Later in this chapter, we give you a selection of classic dishes to choose from whilst dining at your favourite restaurant.

Select plenty of vegetables or salad to accompany your main course. No need to scrimp on the veggies and salad! However, avoid French fries and mashed, roast, and jacket potatoes. If you want rice, pasta, or boiled potatoes, ask for small portions, or request an extra vegetable dish instead. Don't order sticky white rice.

Dressings on salads and vegetables vary according to the type of restaurant but GL-friendly options include:

- ✔ Freshly ground black pepper

- ✔ Vinegar – try balsamic, red or white wine, or rice vinegar depending on which type of restaurant you're eating in

- ✔ Grated Parmesan cheese

- ✔ Fresh lemon or lime juice

- ✔ Chilli sauce

- ✔ Extra-virgin olive oil

- ✔ French dressing

- ✔ Raspberry vinaigrette

Check out the next section, 'Hold the sauce', for tips about selecting sauces.

Not everything you select from the menu has to be low-GL – eating out is a treat, after all. However, ensure that any portions of moderate- to high-GL foods you choose are kept small to balance out the overall GL of your meal.

Sometimes, restaurants have a better selection of low-GL starters than main courses. If you find yourself faced with this situation, why not order two starters instead of a main course, or ask for a starter in a main-course size?

When the time comes for pudding, skip the high-sugar, high-fat desserts and go for a delicious low-GL alternative. Fresh seasonal fruit is usually available, or choose some strawberries or fresh fruit salad with a little whipped cream or plain ice cream. Alternatively, select some tasty cheese with grapes, celery, and a couple of small oatcakes.

If you fancy a really decadent dessert, give in to temptation and order one portion to share. You'll savour every mouthful.

Hold the sauce

A key tip to successfully dining out the GL-way is to ask the waiting staff for more information about the ingredients of the food they offer, particularly the sauces, which can be very high in GL.

In most places, waiting staff must be very well informed about the contents of the dishes to help customers with special dietary needs, such as nut allergies. Take advantage of this fact by quizzing staff about low-GL substitutions or modifications the chef could make to your order.

Sauces in restaurants are usually made with high-GL ingredients such as refined flour, sugar, cream, butter – or all four! Ask your waiting staff to serve your dish without the sauce, or have it served on the side and use a couple of tablespoons as a dipping sauce. Good quality cuts of meat and fillets of fish taste delicious when simply grilled or baked. Alternatively, ask if you can have a different option with the dish, or if the chef can modify the ingredients when preparing the sauce. Cheese- and tomato-based sauces usually have the lowest GL.

Any dining establishment worth its salt puts you, the customer, first and will try to meet your dietary requests. The more often you ask for low-GL options, the more restaurants will see the demand, and adapt their menu accordingly.

Enjoying a Tipple

For many people, alcohol is another one of life's pleasures, which often goes hand in hand with food and eating out. You don't want to be a party pooper just because you're following a low-GL eating plan. In this section, we share our golden GL rules to making clever choices with alcoholic drinks.

GL-friendly drinks

You can use the following rule as a general guide to choosing GL friendly drinks: The sweeter the drink, the higher the GL. Red wine, dry white wine, and champagne all have a lower GL than sweet white wine. Dry sherry is a better choice than medium or sweet sherry. Avoid sweet liqueurs such as Tia Maria and Baileys, as well as alcopops in any form – they're fizzy fruit-based drinks packed with sugar and a GL through the roof. The GL of cocktails depends on the ingredients. Seek out a dry martini or a bloody mary rather than a pina colada!

Spirits are usually low in GL and using a sugar-free mixer reduces the GL even further. You can try:

- Low-calorie slimline tonic and a slice of lemon in your gin
- Slimline ginger or sugar-free lemonade in your whiskey
- Diet cola in your rum or vodka

Ask for reduced-carbohydrate beer. If the restaurant doesn't stock low-carb beer, your request may prompt them to make it available in the future.

Drinking sensibly

Drinking too much, especially on an empty stomach, can make you forget all your good intentions (and our golden rules) and head for the high-GL sections of the menu. Avoid drinking on an empty stomach in the bar before your table is ready. Choose a slimline mixer and save the alcoholic drinks until you're eating.

Sip your drinks slowly throughout the meal. Alternate alcoholic drinks with water.

Keep a careful eye on how often your glass is refilled so that you can keep within modest levels. In the United States the Dietary Guidelines for Americans advise drinking in moderation up to one drink a day for women and up to two drinks per day for men; a drink is half a pint of normal strength beer or a small glass of wine. The United Kingdom's Department of Health advises safe upper levels of no more than 2–3 units per day for a woman and 3–4 units per day for a man when drinking alcohol. To help you keep track, Table 5-1 gives you a handy at-a-glance guide to the units of alcohol in common restaurant tipples.

Table 5-1 Units of Alcohol in Common Restaurant Drinks

Drink	Serving size	Units
Beer, lager, or cider		
Ordinary strength (3–4% alcohol)	½ pint (284 ml)	1
Export strength (5% alcohol)	½ pint (284 ml)	1.25
Table wine, any type (10–12% alcohol)	1 small glass (125 ml)	1.5
	1 bottle (750 ml)	9
Sprits (40% alcohol)	25 ml measure	1.2
Fortified wines (sherry, port, or aperitifs:15–20% alcohol)	50 ml measure	1
Alcopops (fizzy fruit-based drinks containing 5% alcohol)	Bottle (275 ml)	1.4

Dining Out on Food from Around the World

What's your favourite type of restaurant? Indian, Chinese? Perhaps you love eating Greek food to bring back memories of a wonderful holiday? Or maybe you like going to one of the newer Spanish tapas bars? Too hard to choose?

The good news is that no matter where you fancy dining, you can find wonderful low-GL menu choices to please your palate. A little knowledge about the foods, cooking methods, and ingredients keeps you well-armed against high-GL pitfalls. Climb aboard and hold tight – this section takes you on a round-the-world gastronomic tour, GL-style.

Curry some flavour: Indian food

When deciding on your starter, leave out the deep-fried samosas, bhajis, pakoras, poppadoms, and chutney, and choose a couple of side dishes instead (see our suggestions later on). If you want bread, choose a small chapatti rather than naan. If you need a sauce on the side, ask for cucumber raita, a delicious yogurt-based sauce with mint.

The best low-GL main course choices in an Indian restaurant are based on lamb or chicken, or shellfish such as prawns. Choose sauces made from tomatoes, onions, yogurt, lentils, or peas. The drier style tandoori dishes (baked in a clay oven called a *tandoor*) and chicken tikka are also ideal low-GL choices.

As a rule, most rice-based dishes have a high GL. Accompany your main course with a salad or a vegetable dish instead of rice.

Some ideas for low-GL spicy side dishes include:

- ✔ Brinjal (aubergine)
- ✔ Chana (chickpea)
- ✔ Dahl (lentil curry)
- ✔ Gobi (cauliflower)
- ✔ Matar paneer (peas with soft cheese)
- ✔ Okra (ladies fingers)
- ✔ Saag (spinach)

Oriental options

You can find a fantastic selection of low-GL choices from the Far East. Many dishes are stir-fried, steamed, braised, or marinated. Try stir-fries that contain chicken, duck, beef, pork, prawns, or tofu (soy bean curd). Some bigger establishments serve whole steamed fish such as trout or sea bass in ginger. Most dishes include plenty of vegetables. Make sure that you include some of the following:

- ✔ Bean sprouts
- ✔ Cashews
- ✔ Mushrooms
- ✔ Spring onions
- ✔ Tomato
- ✔ Water chestnuts

Satay dipping sauce, made from peanuts, has a low GL. If you're not sure whether the sauce is loaded with sugar or white flour – be it teriyaki, sweet and sour, or black bean – ask your waiter.

Go easy on the rice and noodles or avoid them all together. The sticky rice often served in oriental restaurants has the highest GL of all types of rice. Avoid deep-fried snacks such as spring rolls, prawn toast, and sticky ribs. Instead, start with a clear hot and sour soup or a miso soup made from fermented soy beans and crispy seaweed. Sometimes, these soups come with added pork, tofu, or prawns.

In Thai restaurants try hot and sour soups such as *tom yum*, which combines Thai fish sauce, lemon, and chilli with seafood or chicken. Thai green curry with chicken or seafood is an excellent low-GL choice bursting with coriander and coconut flavours.

Japanese *sashimi* makes an alternative to sushi and is based on thinly sliced raw fish and seafood. *Sashimi* is served with a garnish of *wasabi* (shredded Japanese horseradish) and soy sauce for dipping.

Picking at the pizzeria

Think Italian and you usually think of pizza and pasta dishes – high-GL choices.

Luckily, Italian starters provide wonderful opportunities for low-GL dining. Examples include:

- Three bean salad
- Salad tricolore (avocado, tomato, and mozzarella)
- Fresh tuna nicoise salad
- Vegetable soup, such as minestrone
- Tuna and white bean salad
- Melon and Parma ham
- Antipasto – a selection of cold Italian cured meats, pickles, and marinated vegetables
- Smoked salmon
- Grilled scallops
- Whitebait
- Marinated calamari or octopus
- Mussels
- Prawns

For your main course, pick grilled meats such as steak, veal, or chicken and serve with cooked vegetable dishes such as ratatouille, or choose a large mixed side salad. Italians also do fantastic fresh fish dishes including baked salmon and trout, grilled swordfish or tuna, and fish stews.

 If you really want pasta, ask for a small or starter-sized portion and request it cooked *al dente* (firm to the bite). As a general rule, remember that the thicker the pasta, the lower the GL. For example, fettuccine has a lower GL than macaroni and other thin types of pasta. Go for wholemeal pasta where you can.

Avoid reheated pasta dishes, such as lasagne or cannelloni, where the pasta has lost all of its bite.

The best sauces to accompany your pasta are those based on tomato, wine, pesto, or cheese that contains meat or seafood for protein. Sauces containing pulses or beans bring the GL of the dish down.

Adding a little Parmesan cheese lowers the GL because the cheese is rich in both protein and fat, which delays the rate of stomach emptying and thereby slows down the digestion of the starch in the pasta.

Going Greek

Greek restaurants typically offer a wealth of low-GL starter and main meal options.

Greek starters make wonderful low-GL options. Select from:

- Tzatziki (yoghurt, garlic, and cucumber)
- Marinated octopus salad
- Hummus (made from chickpeas with a sesame seed paste)
- Fasiola gigandes (giant beans in tomato sauce)
- Melitzanosalata (an aubergine dip)
- Grilled halloumi cheese
- Grilled goats cheese
- Falafel (made from spicy chickpeas)
- Tabouleh (salad made from bulgur wheat)

Ask for your starters to be served with crudités (raw vegetables such as carrots, tomatoes, and peppers) or a small portion of warm pitta bread.

Oven-baked dishes with sauces based on wine, stock, and tomatoes are common in Greek cooking. Ideal low-GL main courses include:

- Souvlaki (lamb marinated in oil, lemon, and herbs)
- Stifado (a rich oven-baked dish of red wine and beef stew)
- Lamb or chicken shish kebabs
- Calamari (grilled fish or squid)

Ask for salad or steamed greens to accompany your main course. Greek salad is a classic low-GL dish of tomatoes, cucumber, onions, olives, and feta cheese.

Munching Mexican

Mad about Mexican? Well, you don't have to miss out on the fun because you're eating low-GL style. Avoid the nachos and potato wedges as a starter, but look out for corn on the cob, or gazpacho (a cold tomato soup). Or, you can order crudités with salsa (chunky tomato and onion dip) or guacamole (creamy avocado). Ceviche is a low-GL starter made from fish or scallops marinated in lime juice.

Mexican restaurants usually have several main courses based on grilled meat, fish, or shellfish, all good low-GL choices. Alternatively, go for chilli con carne, packed with low-GL beans. Chile verdi is a wonderful dish of pork and green chilli. Another good choice is plain cooked chicken wings (ask for them without the BBQ sauce). If you want to be really angelic, pick a salad for a main course, but be wary of the dressing (see the section 'Hold the sauce' earlier in this chapter).

Choose refried beans as a side dish and pico de gallo sauce (tomato, onion, and pepper hot sauce) to accompany your dish.

Avoid enchiladas, chimichangas, burritos, and quesadillas – all high GL. If you fancy fajitas, ask for the filling without the wraps, or have one portion.

Tasty tapas

Tapas, literally 'little saucers of food', are the Spanish form of appetisers. You can pick a selection of tasty little dishes instead of a main course. Tapas are a great way to get a variety of low-GL choices for your meal.

Good low-GL choices are:

- ✔ Albondigas (spicy meatballs)
- ✔ Bacalao (salted cod)
- ✔ Boquerones (anchovies)

- ✔ Calamares (squid)
- ✔ Chicken livers in sherry
- ✔ Cured Spanish hams
- ✔ Grilled garlic jumbo prawns
- ✔ Manchego cheese
- ✔ Marinated seafood salad
- ✔ Roasted almonds
- ✔ Stuffed eggs
- ✔ Vegetable dishes, such as artichoke hearts, olives, marinated mushrooms, peppers, or aubergines

Part III
Morning to Night Recipes

The 5th Wave   By Rich Tennant

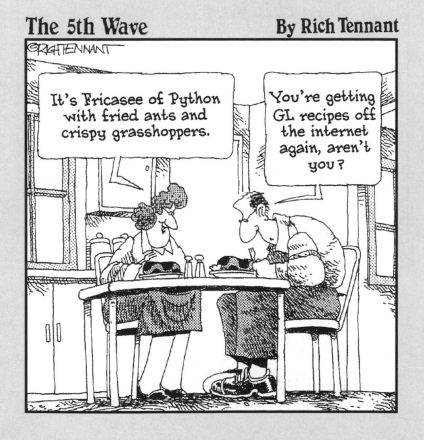

In this part . . .

*P*art III gives you low-GL recipes to suit every meal of the day. We give you some quick and easy dishes and others for when you're in the mood for something a bit more involved. The one aspect all the recipes have in common is that they fit deliciously into a low-GL lifestyle. The word deprivation isn't in our vocabulary!

We use plenty of low-GL fruit, vegetables, and pulses in our recipes to make them full of natural goodness. All the ingredients are readily available. We made the recipes suitable for the whole family, as well as being healthy and tempting to your tastebuds. Whether you're an experienced cook or a novice, we know you'll find something appealing here.

Chapter 6

Starting Your Day with a Low-GL Breakfast

....

In This Chapter

▶ Rustling up traditional breakfasts with a twist

▶ Preparing delicious fruity breakfasts

....

*Y*ou've no doubt heard the saying 'Breakfast like a king'– but did you know that it's true? Breakfast really is the most important meal of the day – so do make time for it. Eating breakfast sets you up to face the challenges of the day (well, until lunchtime rolls around at any rate!). Having something to eat kickstarts your metabolism after a night's fasting, and gives you the fuel you need to operate. After all, you wouldn't expect your car to get very far with no petrol, would you?

People who regularly eat breakfast benefit from having more control over their blood-sugar levels. As a result, breakfasters are better prepared for warding off hunger pangs and are less prone to snacking on high-fat, high-sugar foods such as chocolate bars, crisps, cakes, and biscuits. Breakfast-eaters also tend to concentrate for longer, which can boost their performance, and even suffer less irritability and stress, when compared to those people who skip breakfast.

In this chapter we've put together a variety of low-GL breakfast suggestions to get your day off to a good start. You can find the perfect breakfast for you, whether you've got a lazy morning to indulge yourself, or are dashing out the door and just need to grab a 'breakfast to go'. We guarantee that each of these breakfasts will wake up your taste buds and keep you going until lunch.

Tucking into a Traditional Breakfast

Eating the low-GL way doesn't mean you have to ban sausages and bacon! Enjoy tucking into these traditional breakfasts for when you have a little more time on your hands and can enjoy a bigger breakfast.

Oven-roasted Lazy Morning Breakfast

A great breakfast for when you have time to take it easy. Use high-quality, high-meat-content sausages as some cheaper versions contain rusk and other ingredients, which have a higher GL – ask your local butcher about the selection of delicious herby and spicy sausage varieties available.

Preparation time: 10 minutes

Cooking time: 1 hour

Serves: 2

4 tomatoes, halved

4 lean sausages (minimum 85 per cent meat)

1 teaspoon fresh thyme, chopped (½ teaspoon dried)

1 teaspoon toasted sesame seeds (optional, but delicious)

2 tablespoons olive oil

Seasoning, to taste

2 large free-range eggs

2 pieces low-GL bread

1 Preheat the oven to 180°C, 350°F, Gas Mark 4. Cut the tomatoes in half and place in a baking dish, sprinkle with the thyme and sesame seeds, grind over some black pepper, and then drizzle with olive oil. Gently toss to coat the tomatoes with the mixture, and re-arrange so the seasoned halfs are cut-side up. Add the sausages, lightly cover the baking dish with tinfoil (don't seal it tightly round the edges), and pop into the oven for 45 minutes.

2 Set the timer on the oven, pick up your cup of coffee or tea, and return to bed.

3 45 minutes later, check that the tomatoes and sausages are thoroughly cooked, then lower the oven temperature just enough to keep the dish warm. In a frying-pan heat a small splash of olive oil over a medium setting and fry the eggs until the whites of the eggs are set. Toast the low-GL bread. (Refer to Chapter 4 for what constitutes low-GL bread.)

4 Assemble on a plate and serve with tomato ketchup, black pepper, and a fresh pot of coffee or tea.

Tip: *This dish goes great with scrambled eggs, too.*

Nutrient analysis per serving: *Calories 413; Protein 20g; Carbohydrate 23g; Fat 26g; Saturated fat 6g; Fibre 4g; Sodium 977mg.*

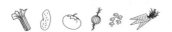

Cinnamon Porridge

This version of porridge has a decadent twist on the traditional recipe. You can omit the milk and replace with a double quantity of water, but it tastes much nicer made with half and half. Fructose is available from most supermarkets.

Preparation and cooking time: 10 minutes

Serves: 2

80g / 3 ounces / half a cup old-fashioned porridge oats (oatmeal)

175ml / 4½ fluid ounces / ½ cup water

175ml / 4½ fluid ounces / ½ cup semi-skimmed (two per cent fat) milk

1 teaspoon ground cinnamon

2 teaspoons fructose or natural fruit sugar

2 tablespoons reduced-fat single (light) cream or Greek-style yoghurt, to serve (optional)

1 Place the oats, water, milk, and cinnamon into a small saucepan and bring to the boil over a high heat, stirring continuously. Then, reduce the heat and simmer, stirring occasionally, until the mixture thickens. You can cook the porridge for up to 10 minutes, depending on your preferred consistency. Add more fluid if you like your porridge runny.

2 Stir in the fructose, and if you're indulging yourself, spoon over the cream or yoghurt.

Tip: Throw in a handful of fresh berries just before serving, or add a handful of frozen berries before cooking; leave out the fructose and drizzle 1 generous teaspoon of honey instead.

Nutrient analysis per serving: *Calories 200; Protein 7; Carbohydrate 35g; Fat 7g; Saturated fat 2.5g; Fibre 3g; Sodium 805mg.*

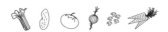

Scrambled Eggs and Smoky Bacon

Nothing is quite as satisfying as bacon and eggs with toast. However, you can reduce the fat content by using only the egg whites instead of whole eggs.

Preparation and cooking time: *15 minutes*

Serves: *2*

6 rashers (strips) smoked lean bacon

4 large free-range eggs

20 grams / 0.5 ounce / 2 teaspoons butter

2 pieces low-GL bread

Seasoning, to taste

1 Heat your grill to medium-hot temperature, and cook the bacon to your preference (some people like crispy bacon, others a little-less well done!). Break the eggs into a bowl, add seasoning, and whisk together well. When the bacon's almost done, place a small saucepan (skillet) over a medium heat, add the butter, and as soon as it's melted, add the eggs. Whilst the eggs are cooking, stir continuously with a wooden spoon.

2 Toast the bread. When your eggs are just done, turn off the heat, then lightly butter the toast, place the eggs on top, add the bacon, and serve.

Tip: You can exchange the bacon for smoked salmon, and grill 2 large, flat mushrooms instead of using toast – mix 1 clove of crushed garlic with 2 tablespoons of butter and spread over the mushrooms. Place under a hot grill (broiler) for a couple of minutes, and when ready, top with the scrambled egg.

Nutrient analysis per serving: *Calories 395; Protein 30g; Carbohydrate 12g; Fat 25g; Saturated fat 11g; Fibre 2g; Sodium 1783mg.*

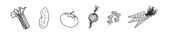

Fast Muesli

You can use any combination of low-GL fresh or dried fruits and your favourite seeds or nuts in this delicious breakfast.

Preparation and cooking time: *7 minutes*

Serves: *1*

1 handful / ¼ cup old-fashioned porridge oats

1 tablespoon raw sunflower seeds

1 tablespoon linseeds / flaxseeds

1 tablespoon crushed walnuts

½ teaspoon ground cinnamon

2 tablespoons dried apricots, chopped

150 grams / 5.5 ounces / ⅔ cup plain bio or Greek-style yoghurt

1 teaspoon honey (preferably runny)

1 Put the oats, seeds, walnuts, and ground cinnamon into a non-oiled frying-pan and place over a medium-high heat. Keep stirring the ingredients in the pan for about 3 minutes – don't let them burn!

2 Once ready, transfer the dry-roasted oats and seeds into a bowl, scatter with the apricots, dollop on the yoghurt, drizzle over the honey, and enjoy.

Tip: Add unsweetened desiccated coconut to the toasting mix for that tropical feel.

Nutrient analysis per serving: *Calories 400; Protein 15g; Carbohydrate 35g; Fat 20g; Saturated fat 3g; Fibre 4g; Sodium 130mg.*

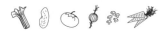

Cheese-and-Tomato Open Toasty

This breakfast is a fairly quick but tasty snack that you can prepare from a combination of ingredients readily available in your cupboard and fridge.

Preparation and cooking time: 10 minutes

Serves: 2

2 slices low-GL bread, toasted

Butter, for spreading

Yeast or vegetable extract, such as Marmite

2 medium tomatoes, thinly sliced

40 grams / 1 ounce / 1 tablespoon cheddar cheese, grated

Black pepper

Basil leaves, to garnish

1 Preheat the grill (broiler) so that it's very hot. Spread the toast thinly with butter and Marmite, arrange the tomato slices on top, and place under the grill for a couple of minutes, until hot.

2 Remove from the grill, sprinkle with the grated cheese, grind over some fresh black pepper, and pop back under the grill until the cheese is bubbling. Serve with torn basil leaves.

Tip: You can use Gentleman's Relish instead of Marmite, if you prefer.

Nutrient analysis per serving: *Calories 197; Protein 8g; Carbohydrate 15g; Fat 12g; Saturated fat 7g; Fibre 2.5g; Sodium 343mg.*

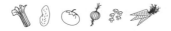

Fancying a Fruity Breakfast

You'll love starting your day with these light and delicious breakfasts. These recipes are jam-packed with goodness.

Continental Breakfast

For this breakfast you can use any low-GL fruit with your favourite cheese and choice of cold meats.

Preparation time: *5 minutes*

Serves: *1*

3 honeydew melon slices about half an inch thick

1 slice cheddar cheese

1 slice good quality ham

4 strawberries

Handful (quarter of a cup) of blueberries

Arrange all the ingredients on a plate, and dig in. Yum!

Nutrient analysis per serving: *Calories 177; Protein 12g; Carbohydrate 13g; Fat 9g; Saturated fat 5g; Fibre 3g; Sodium 545mg.*

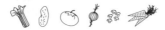

Breakfast Smoothie

You can use any low-GL fresh fruit you like in this quick recipe. As an alternative, you can use frozen summer berries, which gives you a colder, thicker smoothie. Allow the frozen fruit to soften slightly before whizzing.

Preparation time: *5 minutes*

Serves: *1*

1 small firm banana

1 nectarine

Handful (quarter of a cup) of blueberries

150 grams / 5.5 ounces / two-thirds of a cup plain bio or Greek-style yoghurt

125 millilitres / 4.5 fluid ounces / half a cup water

1 teaspoon honey (preferably runny)

1 teaspoon grated fresh ginger

Put all the ingredients into a blender and whizz until smooth and creamy. Drink immediately.

Tip: For a little more protein you can add a measure of vanilla soya or whey protein, which are available from health-food shops (simply follow the directions on the pack for how much to use).

Nutrient analysis per serving: *Calories 295; Protein 11g; Carbohydrate 60g; Fat 2g; Saturated fat 1g; Fibre 4g; Sodium 130mg.*

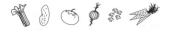

Breakfast to Go

This breakfast suggestion really is a case of grab and go, so you have no excuse for missing breakfast if you're in a rush. Oatcakes come in coarse- and fine-texture varieties, so try both to see which you prefer.

Preparation time: *2 minutes*

Serves: *1*

2 oatcakes	*1 apple*
1 slice of cheese	*Handful of grapes*

Chuck everything into bag and eat as you go. If you have time, break the slice of cheese in half, pop the cheese on the oatcakes, and slice the apple on top.

Tip: Wrap the oatcakes separately in clingfilm to keep them from getting soggy.

Nutrient analysis per serving: *Calories 316; Protein 9g; Carbohydrate 46g; Fat 11g; Saturated fat 5g; Fibre 3g; Sodium 460mg.*

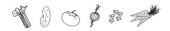

Fruit Salad

This recipe is a refreshing variation on a conventional fruit salad. You can use any combination of fresh fruit that's currently in season.

Preparation time: *10 minutes*

Serves: *2*

Handful / ¼ cup of grapes

Handful / ¼ cup of blueberries

1 apple, cored and chopped into chunks

1 small carrot, washed, peeled, and grated

Zest of 1 lemon

Juice of ½ lemon

1 teaspoon honey (preferably runny)

150–200 grams / 5.5–7 ounces / ⅔ to 1 cup of low-fat yoghurt

Handful (2 tablespoons) of fresh mint, chopped finely

Combine the fruits and carrots, add the zest and lemon juice, drizzle with honey, and mix to combine. Add mixture over the yoghurt and garnish liberally with mint.

Nutrient analysis per serving: *Calories 148; Protein 6g; Carbohydrate 30g; Fat 1g; Saturated fat 0.5g; Fibre 4g; Sodium 87mg.*

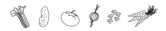

Apple and Honey Nut Crunch

This 'crunch and run' breakfast can keep you energised well into the morning.

Preparation time: *5 minutes*

Serves: *1*

½ teaspoon honey (preferably runny)

1 crunchy apple, grated

1 teaspoon crunchy peanut butter (no sugar added)

1 piece low-GL bread, toasted

Simply mix the honey, grated apple, and peanut butter together, and spread on toast. Delicious!

Nutrient analysis per serving: *Calories 212; Protein 6g; Carbohydrate 35g; Fat 6g; Saturated fat 1g; Fibre 5g; Sodium 205mg.*

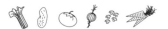

Chapter 7

Doing Lunch: Low-GL Lunches at Home and on the Go

In This Chapter

▶ Boxing clever with packed lunches

▶ Dishing up delicious lunches to eat at home

*I*n this chapter we take out all the hard work of coming up with ideas for lunch. Packing your own lunch is cheap and simple, so we did some 'thinking outside the lunch box' and devised some tasty and easy suggestions for lunches on the run. Eating a packed lunch is not only a great way to ensure that you find a healthy choice at lunchtime, but preparing lunch yourself can also save you money. Making your own lunch takes very little time – just give it a try for a couple of weeks and you may be surprised. Simply add some fruit or yoghurt as a dessert and hey presto – lunch in a box, in a jiffy!

We also include ten satisfying, but quick recipes for when you lunch at home. Tickle your taste buds by serving up Mediterranean Bacon Pasta, or Tomato and Fresh Herb Soup. Enjoy!

Lunches in a Box

Lunch on the run often means fattening up on fast food, scrambling to the sandwich shop, or missing out altogether. Preparing lunch to take with you while you're out and about can seem like a tall order, so we've put together some really tasty, nutritious, and – best of all – quick lunches that you can throw in a box. Some you can even prepare the night before, so you can spend a few extra precious minutes in bed in the morning!

Tomato and Butter Bean Salad

Simplicity itself, this quick salad has a great range of textures and flavours. The butter beans fill you up and the dressing adds a touch of sharpness to keep you on your toes. The salad is great as a side dish with hot or cold meats.

Preparation time: *15 minutes*

Serves: *2 as main dish*

400 grams / 15 ounces (usually 1 tin) butter beans, drained and rinsed

4 large tomatoes, chunkily chopped

1 bunch spring onions (scallions), finely chopped

Flat-leaf parsley, generous bunch, finely chopped

For the dressing:

2 teaspoons wholegrain mustard

1 garlic clove, grated or crushed

1 tablespoon balsamic vinegar

2 tablespoons extra-virgin olive oil

Squeeze of fresh lemon juice

Seasoning, to taste

Put the beans, tomatoes, onions, and parsley in a large bowl. Whisk the dressing ingredients together, pour over the salad, toss well, and serve.

Variation: You can add coriander (cilantro) and basil to the parsley; use smoked garlic; and add a tin of sardines, mackerel, or tuna to make a more chunky salad suitable for a main course.

Tip: *If using raw garlic is too strong or too antisocial for you, then warm the olive oil in a small pan over a low heat, add sliced garlic to infuse for about 5 minutes, then remove the garlic from the oil (discarding the garlic) and mix the dressing together as stated above. Alternatively, you can substitute the olive oil and garlic for olive oil that has already been infused with garlic or other herbs or spices.*

Nutrient analysis per serving: *Calories 265; Protein 12g; Carbohydrate 26g; Fat 13g; Saturated fat 2g; Fibre 10g; Sodium 734mg.*

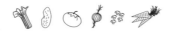

Creamy Tuna Dip

Greek yoghurt works fantastically well with tuna, making a dip with a great fresh taste and a lot less fat than the traditional mayo version.

Preparation time: *5 minutes*

Serves: *1*

1 small crisp apple, quartered and cored

1 can (150 grams / 6 ounces) tuna in brine or water, drained

1 teaspoon wholegrain mustard

2 tablespoons natural, low-fat Greek-style or bio yoghurt

Squeeze of fresh lemon juice

Black pepper, freshly ground

Grate the apple (with the skin on) into a bowl and mix in the tuna, mustard, and yoghurt. Add the juice of about ¼ of a lemon, grind in lots of black pepper, and pop the mixture into a tub for lunch. Eat with carrot sticks and a couple of oatcakes.

Nutrient analysis per serving: *Calories 451; Protein 56g; Carbohydrate 40g; Fat 8g; Saturated fat 1.5g; Fibre 4g; Sodium 1155mg.*

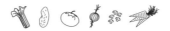

Filled Celery Sticks

Celery is the perfect container for these fillings, and keeps crisp and fresh through the morning. Kids love them too, so these are also great to try when you're all at home.

Preparation time: *5 minutes*

Serves: *1*

4 celery sticks

Fill your celery sticks with any of the following choices, wrap in cling film, and munch merrily at your desk:

a. 2 tablespoons reduced-fat soft cheese mashed together with lots of freshly ground black pepper

b. 2 tablespoons crunchy peanut butter (with no added sugar)

c. 1 small tin sardines in tomato sauce mashed up in a bowl with a squeeze of fresh lemon juice and a dash of Worcestershire sauce

d. 2 tablespoons hummus

Variation: *You can use any low-GL dip that you desire to fill your celery sticks. Try other nut butters, fish pates, reduced-fat herbed cream cheeses, soft cheeses such as goat's cheese, or savoury yoghurt dips such as tzatziki.*

Nutrient analysis (for a.) per serving: *Calories 150; Protein 8g; Carbohydrate 5g; Fat 10g; Saturated fat 5g; Fibre 1g; Sodium 85mg.*

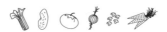

Vitality Salad

Avocado is a great extra ingredient in this salad, but it does quickly discolour. Add diced avocado just before eating the salad, or keep the avocado pieces in a separate pot and squeeze some fresh lemon juice over them, which helps prevent the browning process.

Preparation time: *10 minutes*

Serves: *1*

Half a head of your favourite crunchy lettuce

1 generous handful basil leaves, or your favourite herb (about ¼ cup)

1 generous handful fresh spinach or watercress (about 1 cup)

1 carrot, coarsely grated

1 tablespoon raw sunflower seeds, lightly toasted (dry-fried in a hot pan)

1 tablespoon pine nuts, lightly toasted (dry-fried with the sunflower seeds)

40 grams / 1.5 ounces reduced-fat mature cheddar, coarsely grated (about 3 slices)

1 handful sprouted seeds (available from loads of stores in the chilled section, or sprout your own)

Your choice of dressing, to serve

Shred the lettuce, herbs and spinach, and mix with all the other ingredients. Pour your favourite dressing over the salad, and toss just before eating.

Tip: *To make a fantastic dressing, dilute 1 tablespoon hummus with 2 tablespoons extra-virgin olive oil and 1 tablespoon balsamic vinegar, and shake thoroughly. Voilà – a thick creamy dressing! Alternatively, simply dress with a mixture of fresh lemon juice, balsamic vinegar and extra-virgin olive oil; or use an extra-virgin olive oil that has been infused with herbs or spices.*

Variation: *You can add other greens or vegetables to this fabulous salad, such as broccoli, blanched beans, or rocket.*

Nutrient analysis (without dressing) per serving: *Calories 380; Protein 21g; Carbohydrate 12g; Fat 28g; Saturated fat 6g; Fibre 5g; Sodium 360mg.*

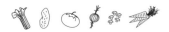

Wacky Wrappings

Lettuce leaves are often used as wraps in Thai cuisine. Firm lettuce such as iceberg works best, although Chinese leaves are great too.

Preparation time: *10–15 minutes*

Serves: *1*

4 outer leaves of iceberg lettuce

Wrap the lettuce leaves around any of the following fillings and secure with a cocktail stick for fast snacks without wheat or pastry:

a. 1 tablespoon hummus and 1 tablespoon toasted pine nuts with a pinch of paprika

b. 1 tablespoon grated cheese with 1 teaspoon half-fat or 'light' mayonnaise

c. 1 tablespoon smoked mackerel mashed with Greek-style natural yoghurt or half-fat cream cheese, with lots of freshly ground black pepper and a squeeze of fresh lemon juice

d. 1 generous tablespoon cooked prawns or shrimp mixed with a tea-spoon half-fat mayonnaise and a small squirt of tomato ketchup

Nutrient analysis (for a.) per serving: *Calories 218; Protein 6g; Carbohydrate 6g, Fat 19g; Saturated fat 1g; Fibre 2g, sodium 269mg.*

Zest for lemons

Many recipes call for lemon zest (the yellow outer skin). The outer skin of the lemon holds the aromatic oils, so gives a great flavour to dishes. How do you zest a lemon? You can buy a zester that allows you to simply scrape the outer skin in thin strips. You can also use the fine part of a cheese grater to get the same effect. Simply gently grate the skin away, turning the lemon as you go. Try to avoid going too deep, or you add the white pith to your zest, which gives a bitter flavour.

Adulterated Hummus with Low-GL Bread and Salad

Hummus is one of our favorite dips. Eating hummus is a great way for people who don't like the texture of whole chickpeas to get a good healthy dose of beany nutrition.

Preparation time: *5 minutes*

Serves: *1*

Grab a small pot of hummus (home-made or shop bought), and mix in any or all of the following ingredients:

Chopped black olives

Chopped red pepper

Chopped spring onions

Toasted pine nuts

Prepare your favourite salad and pop it into your lunch box together with your pot of hummus and a slice of low-GL bread or a couple of oatcakes. Dress the salad just before you eat it.

Nutrient analysis per serving: *Calories 350; Protein 12g; Carbohydrate 17g; Fat 22g; Saturated fat 0.5g; Fibre 4g, Sodium 900mg.*

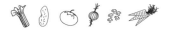

Magnificent Meatballs

This recipe is lean and mean and makes either meatballs or burgers, depending on how you shape the patties. You can add a little more chilli if you like your burger to have a real kick.

Preparation time: *10 minutes*

Cooking time: *10 minutes*

Serves: *2 (makes 4 burgers)*

1 onion, cut into quarters

2 cloves garlic, peeled

1 teaspoon freshly ground black pepper

1 pinch chilli powder

450 grams / 16 ounces minced (ground) chicken or turkey

Zest of 1 lemon

Juice of half a lemon

Small handful fresh tarragon

2 tablespoons extra-virgin olive oil, for frying

1 Place the onion, garlic, pepper, and chilli powder into a food processor and chop the mixture finely. Add the lemon zest and juice and tarragon and 'pulse' until well mixed. Stir the mixture into the chicken or turkey and mix well.

2 Form the mixture into meatballs or small burgers, then heat the olive oil and fry the meatballs over a medium heat for about ten minutes (or longer if your meatballs are bigger) until golden brown, turning frequently. Allow to cool, and then refrigerate.

Tip: *Serve with hummus and salad in wholemeal pitta pockets; or eat with a big salad, dressed at the last minute; or use as a handy snack with Mediterranean-style dips, such as tzatziki, salsa, or guacamole.*

Nutrient analysis per serving: *Calories 275; Protein 50g; Carbohydrate 7g; Fat 5g; Saturated fat 1.5g; Fibre 1g; Sodium 124mg.*

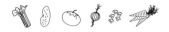

French Bean Salad

Sundried tomatoes have a deliciously intense flavour and work really well with the crisp beans in this recipe. This dish is also a great accompaniment to barbecued chicken or fish.

Preparation time: *5 minutes*

Cooking time: *3 minutes*

Serves: *1*

1 handful fresh French beans, topped and tailed

1 handful fresh spinach or rocket (arugula)

6 sundried tomatoes in oil or dried, roughly chopped

1 handful basil leaves, or your favourite fresh herb

1 tablespoon fresh chives, chopped

1 tablespoon pine nuts, for toasting

1 teaspoon sesame seeds, for toasting

Generous squeeze of fresh lemon juice

2 tablespoons extra-virgin olive oil

1 teaspoon balsamic vinegar

Seasoning, to taste

1 Blanch the beans in boiling water for a maximum of 1 minute, drain, and run under cold water to stop the cooking process.

2 Toss the spinach, tomatoes, basil, and chives with the beans and pop into a lunch box.

3 Lightly toast the pine nuts and sesame seeds in a dry pan, stirring continuously to stop them from burning, then allow to cool, and put them into a twist of clingfilm or sandwich bag.

4 Mix the lemon juice, extra-virgin olive oil, vinegar, and seasoning in a small jar. When you're ready to eat, toss the salad with the dressing, sprinkle over the seeds, eat and enjoy.

Variation: *You can add an avocado, or a can of tuna or sardines just before eating; or add smoked fish or meat. For the dressing, use some of the oil from the sundried tomato jar; use an olive oil infused with herbs or spices; or use a herb or raspberry vinegar.*

Nutrient analysis per serving: *Calories 353; Protein 8g; Carbohydrate 14g; Fat 29g; Saturated fat 3g; Fibre 6g; Sodium 100 mg.*

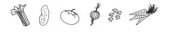

Bacon and Butter Bean Soup

Beans and bacon are a marriage made in heaven. Keep this soup hot in a thermos, or simply zap it in the microwave when you're ready to eat.

Preparation time: *5 minutes*

Cooking time: *30 minutes*

Serves: *2*

400 grams / 15 ounces (usually 1 can) butter beans, drained and rinsed

2 tablespoon extra-virgin olive oil

1 large onion, chopped

6 rashers (strips) smoked back bacon, cut into chunks

4 cloves garlic, chopped

1 teaspoon fresh or dried thyme

1 tablespoon white wine

750 millitlires / 3 ¼ cups chicken or vegetable stock

¼ teaspoon hot chilli powder or flakes

Plenty of freshly ground black pepper

2 tablespoons Greek-style yoghurt or low-fat crème fraîche, for serving (optional, but decadent tasting)

1 teaspoon wholegrain mustard, for serving (optional)

1 tablespoon pine nuts, lightly toasted

1 Heat the olive oil in a medium-size saucepan, add the onions and bacon, and cook over a medium heat until the mixture is just starting to brown. Then pour in the butter beans and garlic, and stir in the thyme.

2 Deglaze the pan by adding the white wine and a little of stock to the bacon and bean mix, scraping all the nice brown bits off the bottom of the pan, then add the rest of the stock and the chilli. Bring to the boil, then simmer the mixture for about 10–15 minutes, keeping the pan uncovered.

3 Ladle the mixture in a liquidiser or food processor and blend until smooth (if you like some chunky bits in your soup, only liquidise about ⅔ of the mix). Return the soup to the pan, check the seasoning, then turn the heat to the lowest setting and let the soup cook for another 5 minutes.

4 If you're going to indulge yourself, mix the yoghurt or crème fraîche and the mustard together. Pour the soup into a thermos flask, wrap the toasted pine nuts in a twist of clingfilm, and spoon the mustard cream into a little pot. When you serve the soup, stir in a tablespoon of the mustard cream and scatter with toasted pine nuts.

Variation: Smoked garlic is wonderful in this recipe instead of normal garlic. You can also stir in some chopped fresh herbs – basil, mint, chives– at the last minute.

Tip: You can freeze batches of this soup to take for packed lunches. Leave a portion out to defrost over night and then reheat the soup in the microwave at work – you'll be the envy of your colleagues during those rainy lunch hours.

Nutrient analysis per serving: Calories 490; Protein 30g; Carbohydrate 28g; Fat 28g; Saturated fat 6g; Fibre 8g; Sodium 1600mg.

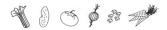

Greek Style Salad

This salad, inspired by tasty Greek food, is lovely with hummus and some low-GL bread or toast.

Preparation time: 7 minutes

Serves: 1

¼ iceberg lettuce, shredded

2 large tomatoes, cut into chunks

¼ cucumber, peeled and cut into chunks

50 grams / 1.5 ounces / ⅓ cup feta cheese, cut into chunks

1 generous handful of black olives

4 sundried tomatoes in oil, drained and cut roughly

2 canned artichoke hearts, cut roughly

1 generous handful fresh coriander, cut roughly

For the dressing:

1 tablespoon extra-virgin olive oil

Zest of 1 lemon

Juice of ¼ of a lemon

1 tablespoon red wine vinegar

Freshly ground black pepper

Place all the salad ingredients together in a bowl and toss. Combine the olive oil, lemon juice and zest, and vinegar in a small jar, with black pepper to taste. When you're ready to eat the salad, shake the dressing together, pour over the salad, toss and enjoy.

Variation: If you're eating at home, fry some chunks of halloumi cheese in a little olive oil and add to the salad at the last minute instead of the feta.

Nutrient analysis per serving: Calories 500; Protein 19g; Carbohydrate 24g; Fat 36g; Saturated fat 10g; Fibre 10g; Sodium 1226mg.

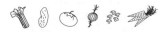

Glazing over

Deglazing simply means adding a little acidic liquid (such as wine, lemon juice, or vinegar) to a hot pan that has previously had foods cooked in oils. Deglazing helps to maintain the flavour left behind by the other ingredients.

Lunches for Home

Just because you're at home for lunch, you probably don't want to spend hours preparing your feast. The good news is that you don't have to. This section gives you more great and speedy lunchtime recipes for you and all the family.

Oven Baked Ratatouille

This ratatouille is delicious with hot and cold meats, or as a main course salad.

This dish tastes great the next day because the flavour intensifies with time. Cook, allow to cool, keep overnight in the fridge, and bring back up to room temperature before serving – ratatouille is tasty hot or cold.

Preparation time: *10 minutes*

Cooking time: *30 minutes*

Serves: *4*

1 large aubergine (eggplant), cubed

2 red or white onions, sliced thinly

2 courgettes (zucchini), sliced

4 large tomatoes, cut into rough quarters

4 tablespoon extra-virgin olive oil

Freshly ground black pepper

1 400-gram / 14-ounce can chopped tomatoes

3 sticks celery, chopped

2 cloves garlic, grated or crushed

2 anchovies in oil, drained and chopped finely (or 1 teaspoon anchovy paste)

100 grams / 3.5 ounces pitted black olives, chopped roughly

2 tablespoons capers, drained

2 tablespoons pumpkin seeds, lightly toasted

Parmesan cheese, grated

Seasoning, to taste

1 Preheat the oven to 220°C, 425°F, Gas Mark 7. Toss the aubergine, onions, courgettes, and tomatoes in the olive oil, and season generously with black pepper. Spread thinly over a large baking tray, and bake for approx 30 minutes, until the vegetables start to brown and get a little crispy round the edges.

2 Empty the can of tomatoes into a medium saucepan, add the celery, garlic, anchovies, and a generous seasoning of black pepper, bring to the boil and then turn the heat down.

3 Stir in the olives and capers to the tomato mix. Remove the baked vegetables from the oven, and pour the tomato mixture over the veggies, mixing together well. Sprinkle the ratatouille with toasted pumpkin seeds and grated parmesan.

Tip: *Add a pinch of hot chilli flakes or powder to the tomato sauce to spice it up; or chop a few sundried tomatoes into the tomato sauce.*

Nutrient analysis per serving: *Calories 256; Protein 6g; Carbohydrate 16g; Fat 18g; Saturated fat 2.5g; Fibre 6g; Sodium 795mg.*

Green Pepper and Nectarine Salad

Don't be nervous about mixing fruit and veggies in the same recipe. Trust us, it works, and after you try it you'll never go back!

Preparation time: *10 minutes*

Cooking time: *20 minutes*

Serves: *2*

1 green pepper, cored and sliced

2 tablespoons extra-virgin olive oil

1 teaspoon fructose or honey

2 nectarines, ripe but not squishy

1 teaspoon cumin seeds

½ teaspoon cayenne pepper

1 teaspoon fresh lemon juice

1 Preheat the oven to 220°C, 425°F, Gas Mark 7.

2 Put the peppers on a shallow roasting tray and drizzle with most of the olive oil and the teaspoon of fructose or honey. Roast in the oven for 20 minutes, taking out and turning once during that time, checking that the peppers don't burn. After roasting, place the peppers on a plate and allow to cool.

3 Remove the stones from the nectarines and cut the flesh into bite-sized chunks. Put the fruit chunks in a salad bowl and mix in the peppers.

4 Toss the cumin seeds in a dry pan until they start to 'pop', but don't let them start to turn brown because they become bitter. Grind the seeds in a pestle and mortar, mix with the cayenne pepper, and sprinkle over the salad. Drizzle over the remaining olive oil with the lemon juice, and stir together.

Tip: *Serve with couscous or low-GL toast or with cold meats or slices of robust-flavoured cheese. You can use a flavoured olive oil.*

Nutrient analysis per serving: *Calories 161; Protein 2g; Carbohydrate 14g; Fat 11g; Saturated fat 2g; Fibre 2.5g; Sodium 4mg.*

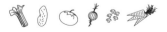

Bean and Green Salad with Tomatoes

This salad is so full of texture and flavour that your senses are in for the time of their lives. Eat as a light lunch, or add a soft poached egg for a sophisticated supper.

Preparation time: 10 minutes

Cooking time: 10 minutes

Serves: 2

1 tablespoon extra-virgin olive oil

1 red onion, sliced

2 cloves garlic, crushed or grated

2 rashers (strips) lean smoky bacon, cut into chunks

400 grams / 15 ounces haricot beans (cut green beans) (usually 1 can), drained and rinsed

4 plum tomatoes, cut into quarters

1 small courgette (zucchini), washed and coarsely grated

2 large handfuls spinach

2 large handfuls rocket (arugula) or watercress

1 tablespoon extra-virgin olive oil, for serving

Juice of ½ a lemon

Generous handful fresh coriander (cilantro), roughly chopped

1 Heat the olive oil in a large frying pan over a medium heat, add the sliced onion, and cook for a few minutes. Add the garlic and bacon. When the bacon is browning, add the haricot beans and tomatoes.

2 Place the leaves and grated courgette into a large salad bowl, and add the warm bean mix. Pour over the extra-virgin olive oil and the lemon juice, toss vigorously to mix and to wilt the leaves a little, and sprinkle with the fresh coriander.

Variation: You can use 50 grams of spicy sausage such as chorizo instead of bacon; use chopped sundried tomatoes and their oil for the dressing in place of fresh tomatoes out of season; and you can use other pulses such as chickpeas in place of the haricot beans.

Nutrient analysis per serving: Calories 218; Protein 10g; Carbohydrate 13g; Fat 14g; Saturated fat 2.5g; Fibre 4g; Sodium 541mg.

Chicken and Vegetable Crumble

This crumble is perfect for those chilly days when you really want to eat for comfort. The oats in the crumble topping give a lovely nutty flavour.

Preparation time: *10 minutes*

Cooking time: *20 minutes*

Serves: *4*

2 tablespoons extra-virgin olive oil

400 grams / 15 ounces chickpeas (usually 1 tin), drained and rinsed

3 large skinless, boneless chicken breasts, cut into chunks

2 garlic cloves, crushed or grated

1 pinch medium-hot chilli powder

2 courgettes (zucchini), washed and julienned (chopped into thin strips)

1 carrot, washed and julienned

400 grams / 14 ounces (usually 1 tin) chopped tomatoes

75 grams / 2.5 ounces / ¼ cup mature reduced-fat cheddar cheese, grated finely

75 grams / 2.5 ounces / ¼ cup porridge oats

1 teaspoon chilli powder

Seasoning, to taste

1 Heat the olive oil in a pan over a medium heat. Cook the chicken pieces until browned (about 10–12 minutes), turning occasionally.

2 Add the chickpeas, garlic, and chilli, and stir for a minute or two. Add the courgette and carrot, and stir for 30 seconds, then add the tomatoes and stir together. Cook for another few minutes until the chicken pieces are no longer pink in the middle and are properly cooked through. Season generously. Transfer to an oven-proof dish.

3 Mix the cheddar, oats, and chilli powder in a bowl and rub together with your fingers to make a savoury crumble. Sprinkle the crumble evenly over the chicken and vegetables mixture, and cook under a hot grill (broiler) until the top is golden.

Tip: *Serve on a bed of spinach, which will wilt deliciously under the hot bake.*

Nutrient analysis per serving: *Calories 425; Protein 41g; Carbohydrate 32g; Fat 16g; Saturated fat 4g; Fibre 6 g; Sodium 270mg.*

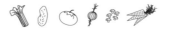

Mediterranean Bacon Pasta

This dish conjures up ideas of a sun-drenched Mediterranean shore-line, and is perfect for a relaxing summer lunch.

Preparation time: *10 minutes*

Cooking time: *10 minutes*

Serves: *4*

200 grams / 7 ounces dried pasta
(penne or fusilli)

2 tablespoon extra-virgin olive oil

6 rashers (strips) of lean bacon, cut
into cubes

1 onion, diced

2 cloves garlic, crushed or grated

400 grams / 15 ounces (usually 1 can)
chickpeas, drained and rinsed

60 grams / 2 ounces sundried
tomatoes, dried, or in oil, drained
chopped roughly

60 grams / 2 ounces pitted black olives,
chopped roughly

Large handful fresh basil, chopped
roughly

Seasoning, to taste

Parmesan, grated for serving

1 Cook the pasta as per the instructions on the packet until al dente (offers a little resistance when you bite it), drain, and rinse with cold water to stop the cooking process.

2 Heat the olive oil in a frying pan, add the bacon and cook for about 2 minutes. Then add the onion and the garlic to the pan. Cook until the bacon starts to brown, stirring occasionally. Stir in the chickpeas, the sundried tomatoes, and the olives.

3 Add the pasta, and stir through to warm. Gently mix in the basil, and serve on warmed plates with plenty of black pepper and parmesan, to taste.

Nutrient analysis per serving: *Calories 474; Protein 24g; Carbohydrate 57g; Fat 18g; Saturated fat 4g; Fibre 7g; Sodium 1136mg.*

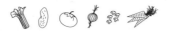

Warm and Smoky Lentil Couscous

This recipe calls for a lot of herbs and spices, but the couscous can take it if you can! The flavours work really well together, especially if you can make it a little in advance.

Preparation time: *10 minutes*

Cooking time: *10 minutes (plus the time for lentils and couscous to cook as per the packet)*

Serves: *4*

4 cardamom pods	*1 red onion, finely diced*	*3 smoked garlic cloves, crushed (if you can't find smoked, normal will do)*
110 grams / 3.5 ounces / ½ cup dried Puy lentils	*4 rashers (strips) lean smoked bacon, cut into chunks*	
110 grams / 3.5 ounces / ½ cup dried couscous		*Generous handful fresh coriander, chopped finely*
1 teaspoon coriander seeds	*1 teaspoon smoked paprika (if you can't find smoked, normal will do)*	
1 teaspoon cumin seeds	*2 anchovies, drained and chopped finely*	*Freshly ground black pepper*
3 tablespoons extra-virgin olive oil		*Lemon wedges and parmesan shavings to serve*

1 Add the cardamom pods to the water that you cook the lentils in and then cook the lentils until tender (about 20 minutes). Rinse and drain.

2 Cook the couscous following the instructions on the packet (usually adding boiled water and leaving to rest for 5 minutes until the water is absorbed).

3 In a large frying pan, dry-fry the coriander seeds and cumin seeds for 30 seconds, stirring all the time, then remove from the pan and crush in a pestle and mortar. Heat the olive oil in the frying pan, add the crushed spices and the onion, stir for a minute or two then add the chunks of bacon. When the onion and bacon mixture is cooked, stir in the lentils (you can leave the cardamom pods in or take them out depending on your taste), couscous, paprika, anchovies, and smoked garlic.

4 Remove the pan from the heat, stir in the fresh coriander, and add plenty of black pepper. Serve with lemon wedges and parmesan shavings.

Variation: You can use 90 grams of bulgur wheat instead of the couscous; use different lentils; use other smoked meats instead of bacon; chop in some sundried tomatoes or red peppers; and sprinkle with a little shaved or grated smoked cheese instead of parmesan.

Nutrient analysis per serving: *Calories 348; Protein 19g; Carbohydrate 38g; Fat 14g; Saturated fat 3.5g; Fibre 4g; Sodium 655mg.*

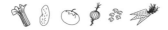

Grilled Goat's Cheese and Salad

Goat's cheese has a wonderfully sharp flavour and stands up well to the robust sundried tomatoes and peppery salad leaves.

Preparation time: *5 minutes*

Cooking time: *15 minutes*

Serves: *2*

2 generous handfuls fresh spinach leaves	*4 sundried tomatoes, drained of oil, chopped into chunks*	*2 tablespoons extra-virgin olive oil*
1 generous handful rocket (arugula)	*100 grams / 3.5 ounces soft goat's cheese with rind*	*1 tablespoon balsamic vinegar*
		Freshly ground black pepper

1 Pre-heat the grill to hot.

2 Divide the spinach, rocket, and sundried tomatoes between two plates, creating an artful base for the goat's cheese.

3 Cut the goat's cheese into rounds, place on foil on the grill pan and grill for a couple of minutes until the top starts to bubble.

4 Arrange the goat's cheese on top of the salad. Drizzle with the olive oil and balsamic vinegar, and grind over lots of black pepper.

Variation: You can use some of the oil that the sundried tomatoes came in as dressing; experiment with other soft cheeses; choose other salad leaves; and add herbs to the salad.

Nutrient analysis per serving: *Calories 314; Protein 11g; Carbohydrate 6g; Fat 27g; Saturated fat 9g; Fibre 3g; Sodium 801mg.*

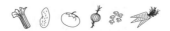

Corned Beef Hash

This recipe is an all-time favourite with a twist. The sweet potatoes make this dish so colourful you won't know whether to eat it or frame it!

Preparation and cooking time: *20 minutes*

Serves: *2*

1 medium-sized sweet potato, chopped into chunks

1 tablespoon butter

2 tablespoon extra-virgin olive oil

1 onion, diced

1 large tin (300g / 10½ ounces) lean corned beef, chopped into chunks

2 cloves garlic, crushed or grated

Dash of Tabasco or other pepper sauce, or pinch of chilli

2 anchovies, drained and chopped finely (or 1 teaspoon anchovy paste)

Seasoning, to taste

Fresh chives, chopped finely

Mixed salad leaves, low-fat mayonnaise, and lemon wedges, to serve

1 Boil a pan of water and cook the chunks of sweet potato for about 10 minutes, then drain and mash roughly, adding a generous tablespoon of butter.

2 In a frying pan, heat the olive oil and fry the onion over a medium heat. When the onion starts to brown, add the corned beef, garlic, and sweet potato mash to the pan and mix together.

3 Add the Tabasco sauce and the anchovies, mix together, and allow to cook for about 5–7 minutes until the mixture starts to brown.

4 Taste and adjust seasoning if necessary (be careful – the mixture is hot!), take off the heat, sprinkle with fresh chives, and serve with a crisp salad, lemon wedges, and a dollop of low-fat mayonnaise.

Variation: *Why not chop in some sundried tomatoes? Add a couple of teaspoons of mustard instead of the pepper sauce or chilli; experiment with other herbs.*

Nutrient analysis per serving: Calories 570; Protein 40g, Carbohydrate 28g; Fat 30g; Saturated fat 12g; Fibre 2g; Sodium 1300mg.

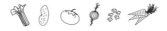

Open BLT with Avocado 'Butter'

Yes, that's right – BLT as a healthy eating recipe! Remember, all foods can be good for you with just a little know-how.

Preparation and cooking time: *5 minutes*

Serves: *2*

2 slices low-GL bread

4 rashers (strips) lean bacon

1 ripe avocado

1 tablespoon fresh lemon juice

1 tablespoon Worcestershire sauce

1 teaspoon Tabasco (pepper) sauce

Handful shredded iceberg lettuce

1 large tomato, sliced

1 Toast the low-GL bread, or if you prefer, don't bother toasting it – your choice. Grill the bacon until cooked, and keep it warm.

2 Take the stone out of the avocado and scoop out the flesh into a bowl. Gently mash in the lemon juice, Worcester sauce, and Tabasco sauce. Spread a thick layer of the avocado 'butter' onto the low-GL bread or toast. Top with the lettuce, tomatoes, and bacon.

Tip: *Serve with a little tomato ketchup!*

Nutrient analysis per serving: Calories 296; Protein 16g; Carbohydrate 16g; Fat 19g; Saturated fat 5g; Fibre 5g; Sodium 821mg.

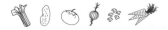

Tomato and Fresh Herb Soup

Fresh is the word with this super easy soup. The herbs and the yoghurt really work together to set your tastebuds singing.

Preparation time: *5 minutes*

Cooking time: *20 minutes*

Serves: *4*

2 tablespoon extra-virgin olive oil

2 large onions, diced

6 cloves of garlic, crushed

1 small glass (50ml) dry sherry

2 x 400-gram / 2 x 14-ounce cans chopped tomatoes

500 millilitres / 2 cups chicken or vegetable stock

1 tablespoon Worcestershire sauce

1 teaspoon Tabasco sauce

3 large handfuls fresh herbs (basil, tarragon, coriander, mint, and so on), roughly chopped

Lashings of freshly ground black pepper

4 tablespoons reduced-fat Greek-style natural yoghurt or low-fat crème fraîche, to serve.

1 Heat the olive oil in a large pan, add the onions, and cook for about 2–3 minutes.

2 Stir in the garlic and then the sherry. Add the tomatoes, stock, Worcester sauce, Tabasco, and most of the herbs (retain enough for scattering decoration), and stir together. Bring to the boil and then simmer for 15–20 minutes.

3 If you prefer smooth tomato soup, take the mixture off the heat and put through a blender. Return to the pan, taste, and adjust seasoning. Alternatively, use the unblended mixture. Serve in bowls with a sprinkling of the herbs, a tablespoon of natural yoghurt, and a slice of low-GL buttered toast each.

Variation: *You can use fresh tomatoes instead of tinned – simply wash and chop into rough chunks, and increase the cooking time to about 30 minutes. You can add more heat with more Tabasco sauce, or use hot chilli powder or flakes.*

Nutrient analysis per serving: Calories 191; Protein 7g; Carbohydrate 17g; Fat 9g; Saturated fat 3g; Fibre 3g; Sodium 512mg.

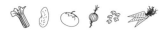

Chapter 8

Delectable Dinners: Low-GL Suppers and Ideas for Entertaining

In This Chapter

▶ Conjuring up quick, healthy dishes

▶ Entertaining in style with dinner-party delights

*A*fter reviewing our favourite low-GL main course recipes, we've hand-picked a selection of 20 delectable dinners that we know you'll enjoy both making and eating. After a long day, you want cooking dinner to be a quick and easy affair, so we've included plenty of nutritious meals that you can make with a minimum of effort, such as Fast Dinner Pizza Pieces for Two. You may want to impress dinner guests with something a little more sophisticated, so why not try dishes such as Stuffed Savoury Crêpes or Roast Chicken with Spicy Yoghurt Sauce, which do take more time and care to prepare, but are guaranteed to deliver maximum wow-factor, low-GL style.

You'll discover something mouth-watering to suit every occasion, from the combined colours of our Roasted Vegetables with Wild Rice, to a new take on an old favourite – Salmon and Sweet Potato Fishcakes. We hope that you enjoy these dinners as much as we do and that they inspire you to come up with ways to adapt your own favourite main-meal recipes, *the GL way.*

Cooking Speedy Suppers to Satisfy

As you can see from the recipes in this section, eating low-GL doesn't reduce your food options at all – you have a wealth of delicious, healthy options to choose from.

Burgers and Mash with Spicy Salsa

Who said burgers were a no-no on a healthy diet? Not us! These little guys wipe the floor with anything you can buy at the drive thru!

Preparation time: *10 minutes*

Cooking time: *20 minutes*

Serves: *4*

For the salsa:

1 onion, cut into chunks

1 clove garlic, peeled

1 pinch chilli powder

Large handful fresh coriander (cilantro)

4 tomatoes, cut into quarters

1 ripe avocado, stoned and cut into thick slices

Juice half a fresh lemon

For the burgers:

1 onion, cut in chunks

2 garlic cloves, peeled

2 tablespoons low-fat crème fraîche

500 grams / 1 pound extra-lean minced (ground) beef

Generous handful fresh coriander (cilantro) (optional)

½ teaspoon ground cardamom seeds (optional)

Freshly ground black pepper, to taste

2 tablespoons extra-virgin olive oil, for frying

For the mash:

2 medium sweet potatoes, peeled cut into chunks

1 onion, sliced finely

1 tablespoon extra-virgin olive-oil, for frying

Fresh salad leaves, to serve

1 Put the onion, chilli, garlic, and coriander in a food processor and blend for 2 or 3 pulses. Add the tomato chunks and blend for 1 or 2 pulses. Spoon into a bowl and stir in the avocado, squeeze over the lemon juice, cover, and refrigerate.

2 In the same food processor (no need to wash it out) put the onion, garlic, and crème fraîche, and blend finely. Add the coriander and cardamom seeds and process on 'pulse' until everything is well chopped and blended. Add the mixture to the ground beef in a bowl, season with black pepper, and stir well. Shape the mixture into 4 burgers and set aside.

3 Boil the sweet potatoes for 12–14 minutes until tender; drain, mash, and keep warm.

4 In a large frying pan, heat 1 tablespoon of the olive oil and cook the onion until slightly browned, then remove from the pan and mix it into the sweet potato mash. Season the mash generously, and keep warm.

5 In the large frying pan, heat 2 tablespoons of olive oil and fry the burgers for about 3 minutes on each side.

6 To assemble, heap a pile of mash on each plate, lean a burger against each pile, spoon over a generous amount of salsa, and season. Serve with a generous portion of fresh salad, dress with a squeeze of lemon juice and some olive oil, and garnish with fresh lemon wedges.

Variation: *You can melt a slice of goat's cheese or your favourite cheese on top of each burger when nearly cooked. Make sweet potato fries, or serve with vegetable mash (cauliflower, celeriac, sweet potato, and so on); or serve with roasted vegetables.*

Nutrient analysis per serving: *Calories 310; Protein 28g; Carbohydrate 15g; Fat 15g; Saturated fat 5g; Fibre 4g; sodium 93mg.*

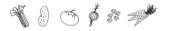

Salmon All-in-One Parcels

Salmon is a naturally rich source of heart friendly omega 3, so we think of these as little parcels made from the heart for the heart!

Preparation time: *10 minutes*

Cooking time: *15–20 minutes*

Serves: *2*

400 grams / 14 ounces (usually 1 tin) flageolet beans, drained and rinsed

1 small jar (150 grams / 5 ounces) marinaded artichoke hearts, drained (reserve 2 tablespoons oil)

100 grams / 3.5 ounces cherry tomatoes, on the vine

2 salmon steaks

Juice and zest of 1 lemon

1 teaspoon wholegrain mustard

1 tablespoon balsamic vinegar (optional)

Freshly ground black pepper, to taste

Lemon wedges, to serve

1 Preheat the oven to 220°C, 425°F, Gas Mark 7. Take four very large lengths of baking foil, fold each sheet in half, and turn up the four edges to make a roomy 'parcel'.

2 Divide the beans and artichokes into each parcel, and top them with the whole tomatoes and salmon steaks.

3 In a bowl, whisk together the lemon juice and zest, oil from the artichoke jar, mustard, and balsamic vinegar, then pour over the salmon parcels, and generously season with black pepper. Close the 'parcels' by pinching the foil together enclosing the salmon steaks, and place on a large baking tray. Bake in the oven for 15–20 minutes until the salmon is tender and the tomatoes are deliciously squishy. Serve with lemon wedges and black pepper.

Variation: *This recipe works with most fish and with other beans, such as butter beans, chickpeas, haricot beans, and even French beans. You can also use a bed of fresh spinach instead of the beans and artichokes.*

Nutrient analysis per serving: *Calories 541; Protein 41g; Carbohydrate 26g; Fat 30g; Saturated fat 5g; Fibre 6g; Sodium 198mg.*

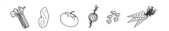

Salmon and Sweet Potato Fishcakes

These fishcakes are great to make in advance or in batches to freeze.

Preparation time: *30 minutes*

Cooking time: *5 minutes*

Serves: *4*

1 large free-range egg

400 grams / 14 ounces sweet potato, cut into chunks

400 grams / 14 ounces salmon (tinned or fresh)

Zest of 1 lemon

1 teaspoon wholegrain mustard

2 tablespoons fresh coriander, finely chopped

Freshly ground black pepper

Extra-virgin olive oil, for frying

Mixed salad or steamed low-GL vegetables, to serve

1 Hard boil the egg in cold water in a small pan. Bring to the boil and simmer for 12 minutes. Immerse in cold water, peel, and chop finely.

2 Meanwhile cook sweet potato chunks for 10–12 minutes until tender, drain well, and mash.

3 If you are using fresh salmon, poach the steak or fillet in a frying pan with just enough water to cook it, then remove from the water and flake the salmon into the sweet potato mash. If you are using tinned salmon, then drain, remove any large bones, and crumble into the sweet potato mash.

4 Mix all the ingredients together well in a large bowl, and form into 4 large fishcakes, or 8 smaller ones. Fry over a medium heat in olive oil, and serve immediately with fresh salad or steamed low-GL vegetables.

Nutrient analysis per serving: *Calories 289; Protein 21g; Carbohydrate 21g; Fat 14g; Saturated fat 3g; Fibre 2.5g; Sodium 192mg.*

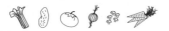

Tuna Pasta Bake

Tuna is a very popular fish that most people enjoy eating. The tuna works well here with a little spice from the horseradish or chilli.

Preparation time: *20 minutes*

Cooking time: *20 minutes*

Serves: *4*

160 grams / 3.5 ounces / 1 cup dried fusilli pasta

2 tablespoons extra-virgin olive oil

2 large onions, sliced

2 x 200 grams / 7 ounce cans tuna in brine, drained

3–6 cloves garlic, crushed or grated (you can use less or more to your taste)

2 teaspoons wholegrain mustard

1 teaspoon horseradish or ½ teaspoon hot chilli flakes

Freshly ground black pepper, to taste

400 grams / 14 ounces (usually 1 can) haricot beans, drained and rinsed

400 grams / 14 ounces (usually 1 can) chopped tomatoes 3 tablespoons half-fat soft cheese or low-fat crème fraîche or natural Greek-style yoghurt

1 low-fat mozzarella block (approximately 150 grams / 3 ounces), cut into cubes

Large handful fresh basil, roughly chopped

50 grams / 1.5 ounces / ¼ cup reduced-fat mature cheddar, grated finely

1 Preheat the oven to 200°C / 400°F / Gas Mark 6. Cook the pasta as per the instructions on the packet, cook until al dente (firm to the bite), drain immediately, and running under cold water to stop the cooking process. Set aside.

2 In a large frying pan, heat the olive oil and soften the onions. Add the tuna and the garlic, then stir in the mustard, the horseradish or chilli, and season generously with black pepper. Stir in the haricot beans and allow to cook for a few minutes. Pour over the chopped tomatoes and stir in the soft cheese (or crème fraîche or yoghurt). Remove from the heat, and stir in the cooked pasta, mozzarella, and basil. Transfer the mixture into a shallow baking dish, sprinkle with the grated cheddar, and grind over some more pepper.

3 Bake in the oven for 15–20 minutes, until the cheese is golden brown on top. Serve with crisp salad.

Variation: You can use sausages (with high lean-meat content), or bacon as a substitute for tuna.

Nutrient analysis per serving: *Calories 548; Protein 47g; Carbohydrate 54g; Fat 17g; Saturated fat 7g; Fibre 8g; Sodium 870 mg.*

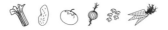

Fast Dinner Pizza Pieces for Two

Try these with a good movie and some fresh salad for healthy indulgence.

Preparation time: *10 minutes*

Cooking time: *4 minutes*

Serves: *2*

2 slices low-GL bread, lightly toasted

2 teaspoons tomato paste

Large handful fresh basil, chopped roughly

Large handful fresh rocket (arugula), chopped roughly

2 slices peppered salami / pepperoni, chopped in half

20 grams / half an ounce Parmesan cheese, grated

40 grams /1 ounce mature cheddar, grated

Freshly ground black pepper

Salad leaves, lemon juice, and extra-virgin olive oil, to serve

1 Preheat the grill to high.

2 Spread the tomato paste on the bread, cover with the fresh basil and rocket, and pop the salami on top of the herbs to keep them under control. Sprinkle with the cheese and grind on lots of black pepper.

3 Grill until bubbling and golden. Serve immediately with more leaves, sprinkled with olive oil and lemon juice.

Nutrient analysis per serving: *Calories 320; Protein 16g; Carbohydrate 16g; Fat 21g; Saturated fat 7g; Fibre 3g, Sodium 700mg.*

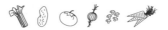

Smoked Fish and White Bean Pasta

Mixing beans with pasta really works well together, as this recipe testifies.

Preparation time: *5 minutes*

Cooking time: *10 minutes*

Serves: *4*

160 grams / 5.5 ounces dried pasta (penne or fusilli)

1 tablespoon extra-virgin olive oil

1 onion, diced

400 grams / 14 ounces (usually 1 tin) haricot beans, drained and rinsed

1 small glass dry white wine

Juice and zest of 1 lemon

1 teaspoon wholegrain mustard (optional)

200 grams / 7 ounces smoked fish, skinned, flaked, and boned (mackerel, trout, salmon)

2 tablespoons low-fat crème fraîche

2 tablespoons semi-skimmed (2 per cent fat) milk

Handful of fresh dill, chopped

Freshly ground black pepper, to taste

Parmesan cheese, to serve (optional)

1 Put a large pan of water on to boil for the pasta.

2 Heat the olive oil in a large frying pan, add the onion, and cook for about 2 minutes. Stir in the haricot beans, then add the white wine and the lemon juice to deglaze the pan. Add the mustard, if you're using, stir well, and let the mixture bubble for 2–3 minutes.

3 Add the pasta to the boiling water and cook as per the packet instructions until firm to the bite.

4 Stir the smoked fish into the sauce, and let it warm through for a couple of minutes.

5 Drain the pasta and place in a warmed serving dish. Take the sauce off the heat, and stir the lemon zest, crème fraîche, milk, and most of the chopped dill, then pour over the pasta. Sprinkle with the remaining dill, and a generous amount of freshly ground black pepper. Add Parmesan cheese, if desired.

Variation: *Stir in a teaspoon of horseradish instead of the mustard; use smoked meats and sundried tomatoes instead of fish; use tinned smoked fish or tuna; use basil, chives, or coriander instead of dill; roast your favourite vegetables in the oven and toss with the pasta and beans instead of using fish.*

Nutrient analysis per serving: *Calories 514; Protein 24g; Carbohydrate 47g; Fat 24g; Saturated fat 7g; Fibre 6g; Sodium 468mg.*

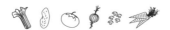

Chunky Spring Soup

This soup is guaranteed to satisfy even the heartiest appetite and every bowlful counts towards those all important daily veggie portions.

Preparation time: *15 minutes*

Cooking time: *40 minutes*

Serves: *4*

2 turnips, peeled and diced

2 celery sticks, diced

2 large carrots, peeled and diced

1 large leek, sliced

2 tablespoons extra-virgin olive oil

2 cloves garlic, diced

1 fresh red chilli, finely diced (or half a

teaspoon chilli flakes or powder)

4 cardamom pods

2 litres / 9 cups chicken or vegetable stock

Freshly ground black pepper

Half a savoy cabbage, finely sliced

410 grams / 14 ounces (usually 1 can)

cannellini beans, drained and rinsed

2 large handfuls spinach leaves, coarsely chopped

50 grams / 1.5 ounces / ½ cup asparagus tips, trimmed

Large handful fresh mint, roughly chopped

Parmesan cheese and crusty bread, to serve

1 In a big saucepan large enough for all the ingredients, warm the olive oil over a medium heat. Fry the turnips, celery, carrots, and leek for a few minutes, stirring well, and then add in the garlic and chilli.

2 Squash the cardamom pods until they split and add to the pan. Pour in the stock, add black pepper, and bring to the boil.

3 Reduce the heat, cover and simmer for about 30 minutes, then add the cabbage and cannellini beans. Cook for 5 minutes, then add the spinach and asparagus.

4 Cook for another couple of minutes, then ladel into bowls, shave over some Parmesan, sprinkle with mint, and serve with crusty low-GL bread.

Tip: *Swirl in a spoonful of natural yoghurt at the end of the cooking process, and add a tablespoon of sprouted seeds such as alfalfa just before serving.*

Nutrient analysis per serving: *Calories 150; Protein 7g; Carbohydrate 12g; Fat 8g; Saturated fat 2g; Fibre 6g, Sodium 261mg.*

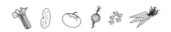

Pea and Sweet Potato Frittata

Frittata is a traditional Spanish omelette dish made with potato. You can put most steamed vegetables into a frittata, but be sure to drain them well. This dish is also delicious cold as a lunch box option.

Preparation time: *30 minutes*

Cooking time: *20 minutes*

Serves: *4*

300 grams / 10 ounces sweet potato, peeled and cut into chunks

2 tablespoons extra-virgin olive oil

1 onion, finely sliced

1 small fennel bulb, thinly sliced

2 garlic cloves, finely chopped

200 grams / 7 ounces frozen peas or petits pois

4 large free-range eggs

50 millilitres / ¼ cup semi-skimmed (2 per cent fat) milk

Freshly ground black pepper

2 teaspoons fresh mint, chopped

25 grams / 1 ounce freshly grated Parmesan cheese

1 Bring a pan of water to the boil and cook the sweet potato chunks for about 10 minutes, until tender but not falling apart. Drain well and set aside.

2 Heat the oil in a medium-sized ovenproof frying pan (suitable to go under the grill, or broiler). Add the onion and fennel and fry until golden. Add the garlic, peas, and sweet potato. Stir gently to coat the vegetables in oil, but try not to break them up. Cook for another 5 minutes. Add the chopped mint.

3 Preheat the grill (broiler) on high. Whisk the eggs and milk together in a bowl with the black pepper, and pour into the pan.

4 Cook the frittata for 3–5 minutes on the hob until just cooked, then sprinkle with the Parmesan and place under the grill until bubbly and golden brown. Serve immediately, cut into chunky wedges, together with a crisp salad.

Nutrient analysis per serving: *Calories 276; Protein 14g; Carbohydrate 25g; Fat 14g, Saturated fat 4g; Fibre 6g; Sodium 247mg.*

Bite-Size TV Dinner Platter

Perfect for a night in or when you need nibbles for guests (simply multiply the ingredients). Make a selection of the ideas below, forget the cutlery, and dive straight in!

Total preparation time: *25 minutes*

Total cooking time: *6 minutes*

Serves: *2*

Egg salad bites

1 slice rye bread, cut into quarters

2 large free-range eggs

1 shallot, finely sliced

1 tablespoon mustard and cress, chopped

1 tablespoon good quality reduced-fat mayonnaise

Extra cress, to serve

Put the eggs in a small pan on the hob (stovetop), bring to the boil, and cook for at least 12 minutes. Run the eggs under cold water to cool, then shell and chop finely. Mix the egg in a bowl with the shallot, mustard and cress, and mayonnaise. Spread the egg-mayonnaise mix equally between the bread quarters, and decorate with a sprinkling of cress.

Spicy avocado spread

1 slice rye bread, cut into quarters

1 small avocado

4 generous dashes Tabasco sauce

1 teaspoon fresh lemon juice

1 teaspoon freshly ground black pepper

Chopped fresh corriander, to serve (optional)

Mash all the ingredients together in a bowl, then spread on the quarters of bread and decorate with coriander.

Hummus and toppings

1 slice rye bread, cut into quarters

1 tablespoon pine nuts, toasted until golden

2 tablespoons hummus

1 teaspoon paprika

1 tablespoon fresh coriander (cilantro), chopped

Spread the hummus equally between the pieces of bread, then sprinkle with the paprika, pine nuts, and coriander.

Salmon and horseradish topper

1 slice rye bread, cut into quarters

1 teaspoon creamed horseradish

2 slices smoked salmon, cut in half

1 teaspoon fresh dill, chopped

Spread the bread with the creamed horseradish, drape with the smoked salmon, and sprinkle with chopped dill.

Arrange all the slices nicely on the serving dish. Serve immediately before the bread goes soggy!

Nutrient analysis per serving: Calories 511; Protein 23g; Carbohydrate 32g; Fat 33g; Saturated fat 5g; Fibre 6g; Sodium 1428mg.

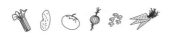

Bake-in-a-Pack Chicken and Vegetables

Kids love unwrapping these parcels, and the aroma means you have clean plates before you know it.

Preparation time: 15 minutes

Cooking time: 40 minutes

Serves: 4

1 onion, sliced	1 small fresh red chilli, deseeded and chopped finely	1 lemon, juiced
2 fennel bulbs, sliced		4 tablespoons dry white wine or dry sherry
400 grams / 14 ounces fresh green beans, topped and tailed	1 teaspoon freshly ground black pepper	Generous handful fresh herbs, roughly chopped, and lemon wedges, to serve
4 cardamom pods	4 garlic cloves, crushed	
4 chicken breasts	4 tablespoon extra-virgin olive oil	

1 Preheat the oven to 200°C / 400°F / Gas Mark 6.

2 Make 4 foil 'parcels' large enough to seal completely when you have the chicken and vegetables inside (like a large foil Cornish pasty!). Use a double thickness by folding the foil in half before shaping it.

3 Divide the onion, fennel, and green beans evenly between the four parcels. Crush the cardamom pods so that they split but the seeds stay inside. Pop a pod in each parcel, and then place one chicken breast on top of each pile of vegetables.

4 Mix the chilli, pepper, garlic, olive oil, lemon juice, and wine together in a bowl, and spoon an equal amount over each chicken breast. Seal the parcels really well so that no steam can escape, and place in the oven for about 45–60 minutes, depending on the size of the chicken breasts. Check they are cooked by making sure the juices run clear when you pierce the breast with a sharp skewer.

5 You can serve the chicken and vegetables in their parcels on plates, making sure that you open them first to let any steam escape. Alternatively, remove from the foil, and serve immediately with fresh herbs and a lemon wedge.

Nutrient analysis per serving: *Calories 305; Protein 27g; Carbohydrate 8g; Fat 16g; Saturated fat 3g; Fibre 4g; Sodium 149mg.*

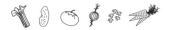

Entertaining Low-GL Style

The recipes in this section are sophisticated dishes for when you need a meal to be impressive as well as delicious and nutritious.

Stuffed Savoury Crêpes

Everyone loves crepes, and these are a great twist on the sweet sugary kind and much better for you.

Preparation time: 10 minutes (plus 30 minutes for batter to rest)

Cooking time: 25 minutes

Serves: 4

For the crêpes:

150 grams / 5 ounces / ⅔ cup stoneground 100 per cent wholemeal flour

25 grams / 1 ounce ground almonds

2 large free-range eggs

150 millilitres / ⅔ cup cold water

150 millilitres / ⅔ cup semi-skimmed (2 per cent fat) milk

1 tablespoon extra-virgin olive oil

1 garlic clove, crushed or grated

2 tablespoons fresh coriander (cilantro), finely chopped (or 1 tablespoon dried)

1 tablespoon extra-virgin olive oil, for frying

For the filling:

1 tablespoon extra-virgin olive oil

1 large red onion, sliced thinly

2 chicken breasts, cut into strips

8 chestnut mushrooms (baby portobello), sliced

400 grams / 15 ounces (usually 1 can) butter beans, drained and rinsed

4 large handfuls fresh spinach

1 pinch hot chilli flakes or powder (or you can use 1 fresh red chilli, deseeded and finely chopped)

50 grams / 2 ounces (half a cup) mature reduced-fat cheddar cheese, finely grated

Freshly ground black pepper, to taste

Fresh salad, to serve

1 Preheat the oven on a low setting to 130°C / 250F° / Gas Mark ½.

2 Make the crêpes first. Mix together the flour, almonds, and eggs. Gradually whisk the water and milk into the mixture to create a nice smooth batter. Stir in 1 tablespoon of the olive oil, the crushed garlic, and the coriander. Leave the mixture to rest for about 30 minutes.

3 Meanwhile prepare the filling. In a large frying pan, heat 1 tablespoon olive oil, and gently soften the onion. Add the chicken strips to the pan with the onion and stir until the chicken is cooked (about 10 minutes). Then add the mushrooms, butter beans, and chilli, and let all the ingredients cook gently, stirring occasionally.

4 In a second frying pan, heat the olive oil and, when hot, pour in enough batter to coat the bottom of the pan evenly. Fry each crêpe for about 2 minutes until the bottom is golden and flip with care – the almonds make this mixture more delicate than usual pancakes – to cook the other side. Keep the cooked crêpes warm in the oven, stacked up on a heat-proof plate, preferably with a sheet of parchment paper between each one.

5 Reheat the filling. While the filling is heating, stir the spinach leaves into the chicken and bean mix. Cook for about 2 minutes, until the spinach is wilted.

6 To assemble the crêpes, place a line of filling along each pancake, sprinkle with a little cheese, and fold over. Serve with fresh salad.

Tip: Make an avocado 'butter' by mashing an avocado with some black pepper and a squeeze of fresh lemon juice and spread this mixture along the middle of the crêpe before adding the hot filling.

Variation: Use the crêpes as lovely desserts filled with fresh low-GL fruit, Greek-style yoghurt, and a sprinkle of fructose or a drizzle of honey.

Nutrient analysis per serving: *Calories 490 ; Protein 35g; Carbohydrate 43 g; Fat 20g; Saturated fat 5 g; Fibre 10 g; Sodium 225 mg.*

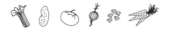

Roasted Vegetables with Wild Rice and Bulgur Wheat

Roasting vegetables is a great way to hold in their flavour and colour, and they make a delicious side dish or a meal in themselves.

Preparation time: *10 minutes*

Cooking time: *20–40 minutes*

Serves: *4*

50 grams / 1.5 ounces / ¼ cup wild rice

150 grams / 5 ounces / ⅔ cup bulgur wheat

Good quality vegetable stock (made from a cube) to cook the bulgur – amount as per instructions on bulgur wheat packet

2 courgettes (zucchini), cut into chunky rounds

2 large tomatoes, cut into quarters

1 large / 2 small fennel bulbs, sliced into chunks

4 whole cloves garlic

Large handful fresh basil, retaining several leaves for serving

3 tablespoon extra-virgin olive oil

Freshly ground black pepper, to taste

Parmesan shavings, to serve

1 Preheat the oven to 220°C / 425F° / Gas Mark 7. Cook the wild rice as per the instructions on the packet – usually boiling for between 30–45 minutes. Drain and set aside. Cook the bulgur wheat as per the packet instructions (usually for 15 minutes), using vegetable stock instead of water. Drain and set aside.

2 Place all of the vegetables into a roasting tin in a single layer – make sure that you don't pile the veggies on top of each other or they will steam rather than roast. Roughly rip the basil and add to the roasting tin, season generously, pour the olive oil over the vegetables and toss, ensuring that they are thoroughly coated. Roast the vegetables for 45–60 minutes – preferably until cooked and slightly browned, not charred.

3 When the rice, bulgur wheat, and veg are cooked, mix together in a large bowl with all the juices from the vegetable pan. Serve onto warm plates, with Parmesan shavings and the extra basil leaves.

Variation: *This meal is also fantastic with the addition of asparagus, lemon, and ready-cooked prawns. Add the asparagus, lemon zest, and prawns about 5 minutes from the end of cooking. Squeeze over the juice of ½ a lemon, stir in some fresh chopped mint, and serve with lemon wedges and lots of black pepper.*

Nutrient analysis per serving: Calories 299; Protein 9g; Carbohydrate 42g; Fat 11g, Saturated fat 2.5g, Fibre 3.5g; Sodium 152mg.

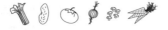

Lowering the GL of pasta

Pasta is a very carb-rich food. But nothing is banned on the GL Diet, so simply follow these tips to lower the GL and tuck in!

✔ Cook your pasta *al dente* (firm to the bite). Overcooked pasta has a much higher GL than pasta cooked just right.

✔ Mix pasta with low-GL beans or pulses such as butter beans, lentils, or chickpeas to reduce the *glycaemic response* (how quickly a food is absorbed into the bloodstream as glucose) of pasta.

✔ Serve your pasta marinara or Bolognese with a large mixed salad – the salad veggies all help to reduce the effect of the pasta.

✔ Don't hold back on the sauce or the Parmesan, because protein foods also slow down the effect of higher GL foods.

Roast Chicken with Spicy Yoghurt Sauce

You can't beat the smell of roast chicken. This dish is a guaranteed winner with all the family.

Preparation: *15 minutes*

Cooking time: *80 minutes*

Serves: *6*

2 medium onions, peeled and cut in half

1 large carrot, sliced

1 large fennel bulb, roughly sliced

3–6 cloves garlic, skinned but leave whole

2 large lemons

1 large free-range chicken, without giblets (cooking times below are based on a 1.5-kilogram / 3-pound chicken)

3 tablespoons extra-virgin olive oil

Freshly ground black pepper, to taste

275 millilitres / 1 ¼ cups cold water

100 millilitres / ½ cup dry white wine or dry sherry

1 teaspoon cumin seeds

1 teaspoon coriander seeds

Pinch cayenne pepper

500 grams / 2 cups natural or low-fat Greek-style yoghurt

2 large free-range eggs

1 Preheat the oven to 220°C / 425°F / Gas Mark 7.

2 Place the onions cut-side down in a baking dish large enough to hold the chicken comfortably, and with high enough sides to hold a good amount of sauce. Add the carrot, fennel slices, and scatter the garlic cloves.

3 Finely grate the peel of one the lemons and set aside, cut both lemons in half and squeeze the juice into a jug. Pop the squeezed lemons into the cavity of the chicken and put the chicken on top of the vegetables in the baking tray. Pour the lemon juice over the chicken, rubbing it into the skin. Then drizzle over the olive oil, and season liberally with black pepper.

4 Pour 200 millilitres of the water and all the wine or sherry into the base of the baking dish, cover the chicken with foil, sealing it well around the edge of the baking dish. Place the dish in the oven and roast for 20 minutes.

5 Turn the oven down a little and cook for another 50 minutes or until the juices run clear when you poke a skewer into the chicken.

6 Gently toast the cumin and coriander seeds in a small dry frying pan for about 30 seconds, then crush the toasted seeds in a pestle and mortar.

7 Whisk the ground spices, yoghurt, eggs, and the rest of the water (75 millilitres) together in a mixing bowl. When the chicken is 15 minutes from the end of cooking, take it out of the oven, remove the foil, and pour over the yoghurt mix. Place the chicken back in the oven for the last 15 minutes, or until the yoghurt sauce has thickened.

8 Take the chicken out of the oven, remove from the pan, and leave to stand to rest for 10 minutes with the foil still in place. Serve the roasted vegetables in a dish and pour the pan juices into a warm gravy boat so that everyone can help themselves. Accompany with freshly steamed low-GL vegetables (see the Cheat Sheet). Sprinkle with freshly chopped coriander (cilantro) if you like.

Variation: *Other great flavours for roasting chicken are garlic, thyme, grated ginger, crushed cardamom, and tarragon. Add to the cavity of the chicken or rub into the skin.*

Nutrient analysis per serving: *Calories 380; Protein 46g; Carbohydrate 12g; Fat 17g; Saturated fat 4.5g; Fibre 2g; Sodium 248mg.*

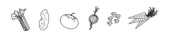

Stir-Fry with Chicken

Stir-fry makes for a super quick and healthy meal. If you prefer, use prawns or fish instead of the chicken.

Preparation time: *10 minutes*

Cooking time: *10 minutes*

Serves: *4*

4 chicken breasts, skinned, boned, and cut into strips

1 tablespoon soy sauce

250 grams / 9 ounces dried noodles – mung bean noodles (these are the lowest GL of the 3), buckwheat noodles, or rice noodles

2 tablespoons avocado oil, coconut oil, or vegetable oil (these oils have a higher 'smoke point' and are better for high-temperature frying)

2 spring onions (scallions), finely sliced

Approximately 600 grams / 20 ounces / 2 to 3 cups fresh vegetables cut into

strips (any combination of carrots, courgettes, baby sweetcorn, mushrooms, bean sprouts, sugar-snap peas, mange tout, sweet peppers, broccoli, cabbage)

2 garlic cloves, crushed or grated

2 tablespoon hoisin sauce

120 millilitres / ½ cup stock – chicken or vegetable

1 teaspoon toasted-sesame oil

2 tablespoons toasted sesame seeds (fry in a dry pan until golden)

1 Place the chicken strips in a bowl, sprinkle with the soy sauce, and toss well, making sure that the strips are coated.

2 Put a pan of water on for the noodles and cook as per the instructions on the packet until *al dente* – you want the noodles to be ready at the same time as the stir-fry, not before, so adjust your timing to the cooking instructions.

3 Heat a wok or large frying pan on a high heat, and swirl in the avocado, coconut, or vegetable oil. Add the chicken immediately and stir-fry for 3 minutes. Carefully remove from the pan, without taking too much of the oil with it, and keep warm.

4 Stir-fry the onion, vegetables (but not the bean sprouts), and garlic (add the garlic last so you don't burn it). Stir-fry for about 2 minutes – until the veg is crisp yet tender. Pour in the stock, then return the chicken to the wok and stir in the hoisin sauce. If you're using bean sprouts, add them at this stage. Return to simmer and stir for about 3 minutes until the chicken is cooked.

5 Drain the noodles, and toss them in the sesame oil and sesame seeds. Serve immediately in warm bowls.

Variation: *To spice up this dish, add a pinch of chilli and Chinese 5-spice or stir in a teaspoon of horseradish for some warm heat. You can use spaghetti for noodles; use Worcestershire sauce in place of soy sauce; and use BBQ or brown sauce in place of hoisin sauce.*

Nutrient analysis per serving: *Calories 533; Protein 42g; Carbohydrate 57g; Fat 16g; Saturated fat 3g; Fibre 10g; Sodium 755mg.*

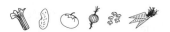

Beef and Bean Stew with Cauliflower and Broccoli Mash

This stew is perfect winter evening fare – make sure that everyone has a spoon for the gravy

Preparation time: *15 minutes*

Cooking time: *3 hours*

Serves: *6*

For the stew:

3 tablespoons extra-virgin olive oil

25 grams / ½ tablespoon butter

2 large onions, sliced

1 kilogram / 2 pounds lean stewing beef, trimmed and cut into cubes

Freshly ground black pepper

2 large carrots, washed and cut into rounds

3–6 cloves garlic, peeled and left whole

10–15 chestnut (baby portobello) mushrooms, cleaned and left whole

200 millilitres / ⅔ cup red wine

100 millilitres / ½ cup cold water

1 teaspoon horseradish

1 teaspoon wholegrain mustard

4 cardamom pods

800 grams / 28 ounces (2 cans) flageolet beans, drained and rinsed

For the mash:

1 cauliflower

1 head of broccoli

3 tablespoons low-fat soft cheese

1 Preheat the oven to 150°C / 300°F / Gas Mark 2.

2 In a large casserole dish (preferably with a close fitting lid), heat the olive oil and butter and fry the onions until they soften. Add the meat and a generous grinding of fresh black pepper. Stir well until the meat is browned.

3 Add in the carrots, garlic, and mushrooms and stir for a minute or so. Pour in half of the red wine and deglaze the pan. Add the rest of the wine and the water. Stir in the horseradish and mustard, crush the cardamom pods so they split – this allows the flavour to disperse – and drop these in.

4 Take the casserole off the heat, put the lid on, and place in the oven for 2 hours. If you don't have a lid for your casserole dish then cover tightly with foil, making sure that it's well sealed. However, if your lid doesn't fit very well, cover the dish with foil first and pop the lid on top – which prevents too much moisture escaping.

5 After 2 hours, remove the stew from the oven, and check the taste (careful – the stew is boiling hot) for seasoning. Stir in the beans. Add a little water if the stew is seems too dry. Put back in the oven for another hour.

6 Cut the broccoli and cauliflower into chunks and steam until tender. Drain well (they retain lots of water), then mash with the soft cheese and plenty of black pepper. You can make the mash slightly ahead of time, just keep it somewhere warm in an ovenproof dish covered with foil.

7 Serve the mash with the stew when ready.

Variation: *This stew works with other robust low-GL vegetables such as swede or celeriac; and other varieties of mushrooms. You can use lamb rather than beef; add a couple of rashers (strips) of smoked bacon cut into chunks for extra flavour; and use different beans – butter beans, haricot beans, and so on.*

Nutrient analysis per serving: *Calories 495; Protein 50g; Carbohydrate 24g; Fat 20g; Saturated fat 7g; Fibre 11g; Sodium 187mg.*

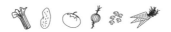

Grilled Lemon Pork Fillet on a Pile of Greens

Pork is a much leaner meat than it used to be, and the fillet is a really tender and succulent cut.

Preparation time: *15 minutes*

Cooking time: *15 minutes*

Serves: *4*

4 lean pork fillets

Juice and zest of 1 lemon

2 teaspoons olive oil

Freshly ground black pepper

200 millilitres / ⅔ cup vegetable stock

1 savoy cabbage, finely sliced

2 tablespoons extra-virgin olive oil

1 teaspoon hot chilli flakes

2 cloves garlic, chopped finely

Butter, lemon wedges, black pepper and some fresh herbs (your choice), to serve

1 Preheat the grill (broiler) to hot.

2 Place the pork fillets in a dish and cover with olive oil, the lemon juice, zest, and black pepper, then leave to stand for 5–10 minutes.

3 Bring the stock to the boil in a large saucepan and add the cabbage. Cover the pan and simmer for 4–5 minutes, at the most. Drain in a large colander and discard stock.

4 Pop the pork fillets under the hot grill and cook for about 3–4 minutes each side until golden and cooked through – exact timing depends on the size of the fillets.

5 Put the saucepan back on the hob, heat the olive oil, and add the chilli flakes and garlic, stir for a minute or so, then add the cabbage and toss in the spicy oil. Take off the heat.

6 Pile the cabbage onto the plates, adding a knob of butter and some freshly ground black pepper, then place a pork fillet on top of each pile, sprinkle with fresh herbs, and serve with lemon wedges.

Variation: This recipe works really well with chicken breasts or lamb chops, too. If you hanker after a 'sauce', fry some mushrooms in olive oil for a few minutes until they soften, add a clove of crushed garlic, deglaze with 2 tablespoons of dry sherry or 1 tablespoon of balsamic vinegar, take off the heat and stir in 4 tablespoons of single cream and a teaspoon of wholegrain mustard.

Nutrient analysis per serving: Calories 320 1, Protein 27g; Carbohydrate 6g; Fat 20 g; Saturated fat 7g; Fibre 3g; Sodium 1 20mg.

Fish Curry with Chickpea Rice

If you're not used to making your own curries from scratch, this is the perfect recipe to start you off.

Preparation time: *15 minutes*

Cooking time: *40 minutes*

Serves: *4*

For the curry:

600 grams / 22 ounces any firm white fish such as cod, halibut, haddock ,or hoki – steaks or fillets, cut into thick chunks

4 tablespoons peanut oil

1 inch piece fresh ginger, finely diced

4 garlic cloves, finely chopped

2 onions, peeled and chopped

1 tablespoon garam masala (or grind together 2 teaspoons coriander seeds, 1 teaspoon cumin seeds, 1 teaspoon fennel seeds, and 4 cloves with 1 teaspoon ground cinnamon)

½ teaspoon hot chilli flakes

1 teaspoon freshly ground black pepper

1 teaspoon turmeric

1 teaspoon cayenne pepper

410 grams / 14 ounces (usually 1 can) chopped tomatoes

200 millilitres / ⅔ cup cold water

Juice of half a fresh lemon

1 fresh fresh red chilli, deseeded and diced

For the chickpea rice:

160 grams / 5 ounces / ⅔ cup uncooked basmati rice

2 tablespoons extra-virgin olive oil

1 onion, chopped

2 garlic cloves, crushed

1 pinch cayenne pepper

410 grams / 15 ounces (usually 1 can) chickpeas, drained and rinsed

Zest of 1 fresh lemon

Generous handful fresh coriander, roughly chopped

Greek-style natural yoghurt, to serve

1 In a large frying pan, heat the oil over a high heat and quick-fry the fish chunks for about 30 seconds. Remove the fish from pan and place on kitchen paper on a plate.

2 Turn the heat down to medium, and add the ginger, garlic, and onions to the pan. Cook until golden, then add the garam masala, chilli, black pepper, turmeric, and cayenne and stir for 30 seconds or so until darkened in colour.

3 Add the tomatoes and the water to the pan, stir, and add the lemon juice. Put the fish gently back into the pan, cover with the sauce, sprinkle with the fresh chilli, and allow to cook for about 10 minutes.

4 Cook the rice as per the instructions on the packet, drain.

5 In a large pan, heat the olive oil over a medium heat and cook the onions until golden, then add the garlic, chickpeas, and rice. Stir-fry for a couple minutes, add the lemon zest and coriander, then serve with the curry and the yoghurt on the side.

Nutrient analysis per serving: Calories 586; Protein 40g; Carbohydrate 60g; Fat 21g; Saturated fat 3g; Fibre 7g, Sodium 170mg.

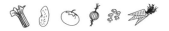

Poached Smoked Haddock with Mustard Mash

We love haddock but you can use any smoked fish you wish for this delish dish.

Preparation time: *15 minutes*

Cooking time: *10 minutes*

Serves: *2*

3 large free-range eggs

1 small cauliflower, chopped into chunks

25 grams / 2 teaspoons butter

2 teaspoons wholegrain mustard

2 smoked haddock fillets

2 teaspoon fresh ground black pepper (or mixed peppercorns, crushed)

2 shallots, sliced into thin rounds

1 garlic clove, finely chopped

250 millilitres / 1 cup semi-skimmed milk (2 per cent fat) and 250 millilitres / 1 cup cold water, mixed

Lemon wedges and chopped chives, to serve

1 Cover the eggs with cold water in a small pan. Bring to the boil and simmer for 12 minutes. Put the pan in the sink and run plenty of cold water over the hard-boiled eggs. Let the eggs sit in the water to cool, then peel, cut into quarters, and set aside.

2 Steam the cauliflower until tender (boil the cauliflower if you don't have a steamer). Drain well, mash with the butter and mustard, cover, and keep warm.

3 Place the haddock fillets in a large frying pan skin side down, and scatter with the shallots, garlic, and pepper. Pour in the milk and water mix (almost covering the fish; if not, simply add a little more water). Bring to the boil, and simmer for about 3–4 minutes until the fish is just cooked.

4 Lift the fish out of the pan and place on warmed plates, scoop out some of the shallot and garlic from the liquid with a slotted spoon to arrange on the fish. Serve immediately with the cauliflower mash, chopped eggs, lemon wedges, and a sprinkling of chopped chives.

Variation: *You can substitute horseradish for mustard in the mash if you prefer. Serve with a crisp salad and a punchy creamy dressing for a lovely summer supper.*

Nutrient analysis per serving: *Calories 475; Protein 50g, Carbohydrate 13g; Fat 23g; Saturated fat 10g; Fibre 3g; Sodium 2112mg.*

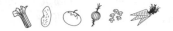

Hot Salad

Hot salads are all the rage, and this is a great, chic dish to serve up to unexpected guests in speedy style.

Preparation time: *20 minutes*

Cooking time: *10 minutes*

Serves: *4–6*

4 tablespoons extra-virgin olive oil

4 chicken breasts, trimmed and sliced into 3 centimetre / 1½ inch wide strips

1 onion, sliced

1 sweet red pepper, sliced thinly

1 garlic clove, crushed

½ teaspoon chilli powder (or 1 small fresh red chilli, deseeded and chopped finely)

1 large iceberg lettuce, shredded

1 large bunch water-cress, chopped roughly

6 large tomatoes, diced

½ cucumber, sliced

1 large avocado, peeled and cut into chunks

Large handful fresh basil, roughly chopped

Zest of 1 lemon

Juice of ½ lemon

1 tablespoon balsamic vinegar

1 In a frying pan, heat the olive oil over a medium heat and add the chicken strips. Cook thoroughly for 10 minutes until no longer pink in the middle, remove from the pan with a slotted spoon (leaving the oil in the pan), and set aside.

2 Add the onion, red pepper, garlic and chilli to the pan, and cook slowly on a low to medium heat for about 5 minutes. Turn up the heat on the pan until the vegetables start sizzling, then add the balsamic vinegar and lemon juice and stir rapidly. Turn off the heat and put to one side.

3 Toss the lettuce, watercress, tomatoes, and cucumber in a large salad bowl. Add the avocado, basil, and lemon zest, and toss again. Add the chicken to the salad, toss, drizzle the hot vegetable dressing over the salad, and serve immediately.

Tip: *Stir a tablespoon of natural yoghurt through the hot dressing when you take it off the heat (it may separate but it tastes delicious and creamy).*

Variation: *You can use any combination of your favourite leaves, herbs, and salad vegetables.*

Nutrient analysis per serving: *Calories 387; Protein 29g, Carbohydrate 13g; Fat 24g; Saturated fat 5g; Fibre 5g; Sodium 128mg.*

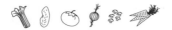

Roast Chicken Pieces with Chilli Greens

If the idea of cabbage sends you running for cover, try our chilli greens – you'll wonder why you never thought of it yourself!

Preparation time: *15 minutes*

Cooking time: *1–1.5 hours*

Serves: *4*

2 onions, sliced chunkily

1 carrot, cut into chunky rounds

4 garlic cloves, peeled

4 cardamom pods

4 tablespoons extra-virgin olive oil

Juice and zest of 1 lemon

1 teaspoon balsamic vinegar

1 teaspoon cayenne pepper

½ teaspoon freshly ground black pepper

8 free-range chicken thighs or 4 whole legs

500 millilitres / 2 cups water, or vegetable or chicken stock

1 savoy cabbage, sliced thinly

1 small fresh red chilli, deseeded and diced (or ½ teaspoon hot chilli flakes)

1 tablespoon extra-virgin olive oil, to serve the cabbage

1 Preheat the oven to 180°C, 350°F, Gas Mark 4.

2 Place the onions, carrot, and garlic cloves into a large baking dish (preferably with a close-fitting lid).

3 Crush the cardamom pods so they split, to let out the flavour. Whisk together the olive oil, lemon juice and zest, balsamic vinegar, cardamom pods, cayenne pepper, and black pepper. Coat the chicken pieces with this mixture and put the chicken on top of the vegetables in the baking dish. Pour any left over mix over the chicken and vegetables.

4 Pour in enough stock or water so that 2–3 centimetres (1 inch) of liquid covers the bottom of the dish. Put the lid on, or cover with foil, making sure that the baking dish is really well-sealed so no steam can escape. Cook for about 1 hour – smaller chicken thighs take about an hour, larger legs can take up to 1½ hours. Check occasionally to make sure that the liquid has not evaporated, and top up with either water or stock if the liquid looks too low.

5 Remove the lid or the foil 15 minutes before the cooking time is up to allow some of the liquid to evaporate and the chicken to brown up more.

6 Steam the cabbage in a big pot, and when just tender, drain well. Set the cabbage aside. Put the olive oil and chilli in the pan and stir for about a minute or two over a medium heat to infuse the oil with the chilli flavour. Pop the cabbage back into the pan and toss well so that the cabbage gets a good covering of chilli oil. Serve immediately with the chicken, vegetable sauce.

Nutrient analysis per serving: Calories 347; Protein 28g; Carbohydrate 14g; Fat 20g; Saturated fat 4g; Fibre 5g; Sodium 96mg.

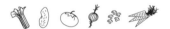

Chapter 9

Just Desserts: Virtuous Low-GL Puddings

In This Chapter

▶ Feeling fruity with fools

▶ Taking a tipple with boozy puds

▶ Getting exotic with tropical treats

Dessert is the perfect end to a meal – especially if, like us, you have a bit of a sweet tooth that just has to be satisfied. Unfortunately, delicious puddings are often packed full of sugar and refined flour. For this chapter, we've wracked our brains, drawn upon our culinary skills, and come up with ten delightful desserts, which fit perfectly into the GL way of eating.

Most of our low-GL puds are based on fruit and yoghurt. However, you need to indulge yourself now and then, so we've included some recipes that use cream or crème fraîche for those occasions when you want to treat yourself. These recipes are higher in fat and saturated fat than everyday puds, so don't say that we didn't warn you!

Creating No-Cook Desserts in a Flash

The recipes in this section are perfect when you want something for 'afters' that's quick and low-GL. Most of these recipes are packed with fruit, so they're crammed with goodness as well as being low-GL.

Squished Boozy Fruit with Creamy Greek Yoghurt

The berries are peachy even without the booze, but a little of what you fancy does you good!

Preparation time: *10 minutes*

Soaking time: *10 minutes*

Serves: *4*

400 grams / 14 ounces / 2 cups
summer berries (fresh or frozen)

1 tablespoon fructose or runny honey

2 tablespoons brandy

500 grams / 18 ounces / 2½ cups
low-fat Greek-style natural yoghurt

Handful toasted almond slivers

1 Squish the berries in a bowl, sprinkle over the fructose or drizzle with honey, and pour in the brandy. Stir together and allow to mingle for about 10 minutes.

2 Spoon the yoghurt into bowls, cover with the boozy fruit, and a sprinkle of toasted almond slivers.

Variation: If you don't have summer berries, lightly cook apples and blackberries with a little fructose and add apple brandy instead. You can use a variety of toasted nuts or seeds, or toasted coconut chips in place of the almonds.

Nutrient analysis per serving: Calories 221; Protein 9g; Carbohydrate 13g; Fat 13g; Saturated fat 7g; Fibre 2 g; Sodium 93mg.

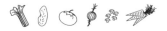

Punchy Fresh Fruit Salad

As well as a scrumptious dessert, this fruit salad makes a great break-fast (without the Cointreau!). Eat the salad with yoghurt or with muesli – or both.

Don't make the fruit salad too far in advance because, even protected by the citrus juice in a covered bowl, the apple and pears can still become a little brown.

Preparation time: *20 minutes*

Serves: *4*

2 nectarines, stoned and cut into chunks

2 pears, cored and cut into chunks

1 punnet (pint) of fresh strawberries, stalks removed and cut in half

1 punnet (pint) fresh blueberries, stalks removed

1 handful seedless grapes

1 apple, cored and cut into chunks

2 oranges, zest and juice

1 lemon, zest and juice

1 small handful fresh mint leaves, taken off the stem and washed

1 tablespoon Cointreau

400 grams / 4 dessertspoons reduced-fat crème fraîche

1 Place the prepared fruit in a large glass serving bowl.

2 Pour the orange and lemon juice over the fruit, and add most of the zest (leaving 1 teaspoon for the cream), the mint leaves, and the Cointreau. Stir well, ensuring that all the fruit is covered with the juice, then cover the bowl with clingfilm.

3 Mix the remaining lemon and orange zest into the crème fraîche and serve it with large spoonfuls of the boozy fruit.

Variation: *Experiment with low-GL fruit combinations; or squeeze over the juice and seeds of a pomegranate instead of one of the oranges.*

Nutrient analysis per serving: *Calories 168; Protein 4g; Carbohydrate 27g; Fat 4.5g; Saturated fat 3g; Fibre 5g; Sodium 20mg.*

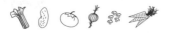

Fruity Cheese Board

You don't have to stick with our cheese suggestions – go wild at the deli and try something you've never heard of before!

Preparation time: 5 minutes

Serves: 4

100 grams / 3.5 ounces Stilton cheese, sliced

100 grams / 3.5 ounces Jarlsberg cheese, sliced

1 bunch grapes, green or red

1 punnet (pint) fresh strawberries

2 ripe pears

8 oatcakes

Arrange all the ingredients stylishly on a serving dish, and dive in.

Variation: Choose your favourite cheese and your favourite low-GL fruit (see the Cheat Sheet); serve with low-GL bread or other low-GL crackers (see Chapter 4).

Nutrient analysis per serving: Calories 361; Protein 15g; Carbohydrate 27g; Fat 22g; Saturated fat 12g; Fibre 2g; Sodium 699mg.

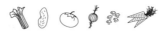

Berry Berry Fool-ish

This dessert is quite high in fat and saturated fat, so only have it occasionally as a special treat!

Preparation time: 10 minutes

Serves: 4

450 grams / 15 ounces summer berries, fresh or frozen (if frozen, defrost first in a sieve over a bowl to remove excess juice)

2 tablespoons fructose, whizzed in a coffee grinder to give the consistency of icing sugar

Zest of 1 lemon

300 millilitres / 1¼ cups whipping cream, well chilled

1 Whizz the berries in a food processor with the powdered fructose. Push the berry mix through a sieve into a mixing bowl to remove the seeds.

2 Add the lemon zest to the berry purée, stir, and set aside.

3 Whip the cream until thick and fold in the berry purée. Spoon into glasses and serve immediately.

Variation: *Try with your own favourite low-GL fruit (see the Cheat Sheet).*

Nutrient analysis per serving: *Calories 348; Protein 3g; Carbohydrate 19g; Fat 29g; Saturated fat 18g; Fibre 2g; Sodium 35mg.*

Zesty Coconut Whip

Like Berry Berry Fool-ish, this dessert is quite high in fat and saturated fat – you have been warned!

Preparation time: *20 minutes*

Chilling time: *1 hour*

Serves: *2*

Juice of ½ a lime

1 tablespoon fructose

1 teaspoon grated fresh ginger

Zest of 1 lime

100 millilitres / half a cup coconut milk (reduced-fat if you can get it)

150 millilitres / ¾ cup whipping cream

1 Stir the fructose into the lime juice until dissolved, then add the ginger and lime zest. Mix the lime syrup into the coconut milk and stir thoroughly.

2 In another bowl, whip the cream until stiff, and fold the two mixtures together. Spoon into glasses and chill for an hour before serving.

Nutrient analysis per serving: *Calories 353; Protein 3g; Carbohydrate 15g; Fat 31g; Saturated fat 20g; Fibre 0g; Sodium 58mg.*

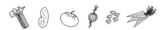

Lemon Ice Ice Baby

A great summertime dessert to cleanse the palate and revive the spirit.

Preparation time: 15 minutes

Freezing time: 2 hours minimum

Serves: 4

2 lemons, juiced and zested

500 grams / 18 ounces / 2½ cups low-fat Greek-style natural yoghurt

240 grams / 9 ounces / 1 cup fructose

Fresh fruit, to serve

1 Put the yoghurt, lemon zest, and fructose into another pan and bring to the boil. Whisk constantly and boil for 2 minutes. Take off the heat and stir in the lemon juice to the mixture.

2 Divide the lemon yoghurt between 4 individual ramekins or ice cream moulds and freeze for at least 2 hours.

3 Remove the frozen yoghurt from the freezer about 10 minutes before serving, and turn onto individual plates. Serve with fresh seasonal berries or other low-GL fruit.

Nutrient analysis per serving: Calories 247; Protein 4g; Carbohydrate 45g; Fat 6g; Saturated fat 4g; Fibre 0g; Sodium 125mg.

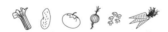

Warming Puddings to Melt in Your Mouth

These special recipes are simply too good to miss. You don't need much time or effort to conjure up impressive desserts for special occasions. Best of all, you don't need to worry about the GL being through the roof!

Grilled Blue Cheese Pears

This combo of pears and blue cheese is just perfect. A real hit with our families and friends.

Preparation time: 5 minutes

Cooking time: 3 minutes

Serves: 2

2 pears, firm and ripe	80 grams / 3 ounces blue cheese, cut into chunks

1 Cut the pears in half, and carefully remove the core with a spoon to create a dip.

2 Cut a sliver off the curve of the back of each half so that the pears lie steady on the plate.

3 Fill the dip first then cover each pear with the blue cheese, and place under a very hot grill (broiler) for a couple of minutes until the cheese bubbles and melts. Serve immediately.

Nutrient analysis per serving: Calories 212; Protein 9g; Carbohydrate 12g; Fat 14g; Saturated fat 9g; Fibre 2.5g; Sodium 376mg.

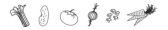

Blackberry and Apple Crumble

The perfect pudding for a cold night. This crumble topping works well on savoury vegetable bakes too if you simply omit the fructose.

Preparation time: *10 minutes*

Cooking time: *30 minutes*

Serves: *2–3*

300 grams / 10 ounces / 1¼ cups blackberries (fresh or frozen)

1 large cooking apple, peeled, cored, and cut into chunks

3 tablespoons cold water

1 tablespoon fructose

For the crumble:

80 grams / 3 ounces / ½ cup old-fashioned porridge oats

40 grams / 1½ ounces ground almonds

30 grams / 1 ounce walnuts, crushed

40 grams / 1½ ounces / 4 teaspoons butter

2 tablespoons fructose

1 tablespoon low-fat Greek-style yoghurt, low fat crème fraîche, or reduced-fat cream, to serve

1 Preheat the oven to 190°C / 375°F / Gas Mark 5.

2 Place the apple in a saucepan with the water and cook rapidly, being careful not to burn them, for about 3–4 minutes. Stir in the blackberries and 1 tablespoon of fructose, and simmer for another couple of minutes. Transfer the fruit to an ovenproof dish and set aside.

3 In a mixing bowl, blend the oats, ground almonds, crushed walnuts, and fructose together. Rub in the butter with your fingertips until you have a nice crumbly texture. Sprinkle the crumble evenly over the fruit, and place in the oven for 30 minutes.

4 Serve with a spoonful of crème fraîche, Greek-style natural yoghurt, or reduced-fat cream.

Variation: *You can experiment with other low-GL fruits; and add different nuts to the crumble.*

Nutrient analysis per serving if serves 3 : Calories 400 ; Protein 7g; Carbohydrate 34 g, Fat 27g; Saturated fat 9g; Fibre 3 g; Sodium 10582mg.

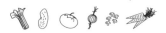

Oven-Cooked Rhubarb with Vanilla Cream

Forget any school dinner memories of mushy rhubarb – this spicy blend goes beautifully with a vanilla cream.

Preparation time: 10 minutes

Cooking time: 30 minutes

Serves: 4

500 grams / 18 ounces / 3 cups rhubarb, chopped into chunks

120 grams / 4 ounces / ¼ cup fructose

4 cardamom pods, split

4 tablespoons double cream

4 tablespoons low-fat Greek-style natural yoghurt

1 teaspoon natural vanilla extract (the best quality you can find, not flavouring)

1 Preheat the oven to 200°C / 400°F / Gas Mark 6.

2 Put the rhubarb and cardamom pods in an ovenproof dish. Sprinkle the fructose over the rhubarb.

3 Cover with the lid or foil (make sure that the dish is sealed well). Cook for 30 minutes, then remove from the oven, uncover, and place somewhere to cool.

4 Mix the cream and yoghurt together with the vanilla extract. Remove the cardamom pods from the rhubarb, and serve hot or cold with the vanilla cream.

Nutrient analysis per serving: 276 calories; Protein 3g; Carbohydrate 35g; Fat 15g; Saturated fat 9g; Fibre 2g; Sodium 66mg.

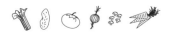

Chocolate Almond Mini Sponges

Light and tasty, these mini sponge cakes are delicious on their own and also go well with any red berries and yoghurt to make a special dessert. Delicious.

Preparation time: *5 minutes*

Cooking time: *20–30 minutes*

Makes: *12 sponges*

50 grams / 1½ ounces fructose

2 egg whites

½ teaspoon vanilla extract

125 grams / 4½ ounces ground almonds

1 dessertspoon cocoa powder

12 split almonds

1 Add the fructose to the egg whites in a bowl and whisk lightly to mix.

2 Stir in the vanilla essence, ground almonds, and cocoa powder, blending thoroughly.

3 Transfer the mixture to a piping bag and pipe 12 small rounds onto a baking sheet lined with greaseproof paper.

4 Place a split almond on top of each cake and bake in a cool oven 150°C / 300°F / Gas Mark 2 for 20–30 minutes. Leave to cool before removing from tray.

Nutrient analysis per cake: *Calories 95; Protein 3g ; Carbohydrate 5 g; Fat 7g; Saturated fat 1 g; Fibre 1g ; Sodium 24 mg.*

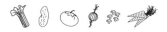

Chapter 10

Smart Snacks: Low-GL Quick Bites and Healthy Nibbles

Don't let the munchies pop up and catch you unprepared. Venture into the world of snacking the low-GL way! Arm yourself with low-GL snacks so that when your energy levels take a dip you don't end up at the vending machine looking for quick-fix foods, such as chocolate, crisps, and sweets.

If you let yourself get too hungry all sorts of unhealthy goodies can easily tempt you. However, healthy snacks can be difficult to find when you're on the run. In this chapter, we provide you with snack suggestions that can fit perfectly into your healthy GL diet to successfully beat your 'between meals' hunger pangs.

You can prepare any of the smart snacks suggested in this chapter in less than 10 minutes. We use ingredients that, with a little pre-planning, you're likely to have to hand in your fridge and cupboard. Head to Chapter 4 where you can find helpful shopping tips for stocking up the perfect GL store cupboard.

We also give you some ideas for small, easily portable snacks in a bag that you can keep handy at your desk, in your bag, or even in the car.

Cold Bites to Rustle Up in a Hurry

These delicious light bites don't even need cooking. What could be simpler? Make a batch of coleslaw or hummus for the fridge so you can dive in when you feel a little peckish. Want a sophisticated treat? Take a look at our snacks on sticks for great appetisers at a drinks party. If time really is of the essence, our snacks in a bag will save you from heading to the nearest chocolate machine, whether you're at work or out and about.

Seedy Coleslaw

This low-GL coleslaw is delicious on low-GL toast, lightly grilled, or in a wrap with some cold chicken or ham. You can also simply scoff it on its own as a scrumptious snack.

Preparation time: *10 minutes*

Serves: *2*

1 unpeeled apple, coarsely grated

1 carrot, coarsely grated

40 grams / 1.5 ounces / ¼ cup reduced-fat mature cheddar, coarsely grated

Large handful fresh parsley, roughly chopped

1 tablespoon sunflower seeds, toasted (dry-fry in a hot pan)

1 tablespoon pumpkin seeds, toasted

1 tablespoon reduced-fat mayonnaise

Freshly ground black pepper

Simply mix all the ingredients together – heavenly!

Nutrient analysis per serving: Calories 250; Protein 10g; Carbohydrate 16g; Fat 16g; Saturated fat 3.5g; Fibre 3.5g; Sodium 183mg.

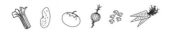

Herby Hummus

This hummus dip lasts for several days in the fridge. Eat it with crudités, oatcakes, or low-GL bread, as a great snack or handy lunch.

Preparation time: *10 min*

Serves: *4 as a dip*

400 grams / 15 ounces (usually 1 can) chickpeas, drained and rinsed

2 tablespoons tahini paste

2 cloves garlic, peeled (optional)

3 tablespoons fresh lemon juice

2 tablespoons fresh coriander (cilantro)

1 tablespoon fresh chives

½ teaspoon paprika

½ teaspoon freshly ground black pepper

3 tablespoons extra-virgin olive oil

Pinch of paprika, to serve

Except for the olive oil, place all of the ingredients in your blender. As the mixture blends together, slowly trickle in the olive oil – the hummus should be smooth and creamy, so you can add some more oil if the consistency is too dry.

Variation: *Experiment with using different herbs such as fresh lemon thyme or even more coriander; and cut down on the garlic if you want to stay social!*

Tip: *Add 1 tablespoon of hummus to your usual salad dressing to make a lovely creamy alternative.*

Nutrient analysis per serving: Calories 230; Protein 8g; Carbohydrate 14g; Fat 16g; Saturated fat 2g; Fibre 4g; Sodium 100mg.

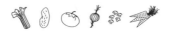

Cold Snacks on Sticks for Healthy Hedonists

These little treats make great, healthy canapés to serve before dinner when you're entertaining.

Avocado, Tomato, and Mozzarella

Preparation and cooking time: *5 minutes*

Makes: *10 canapés*

10 cherry tomatoes

1 ripe avocado chopped into 10 chunks

10 slices buffalo mozzarella

10 fresh basil leaves

2 tablespoons balsamic vinegar

Push a cherry tomato, a chunk of avocado, and a slice of cheese onto a cocktail stick, thread on a basil leaf and drizzle with balsamic vinegar. Easy!

Nutrient analysis per canapé: Calories 63; Protein 3g; Carbohydrate 1g; Fat 5g; Saturated fat 2.5g; Fibre 0.5g; Sodium 200mg.

Watermelon, Feta, and Basil

We can't decide which we love most – the look or the taste of this fantastically fresh combo.

Preparation and cooking time: *5 minutes*

Makes: *10 canapés*

Half a ripe watermelon cut into 10 triangles

10 fresh basil leaves

10 large chunks of feta cheese

Push a triangle of melon onto a cocktail stick, add a chunk of feta, and thread on a basil leaf to garnish.

Nutrient analysis per canapé: Calories 50; Protein 2.5; Carbohydrate 3; Fat 3g; Saturated fat 2g, Fibre 0g; Sodium 217mg.

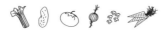

Snacks in a Bag

These super-quick ideas are delicious and nutritious and will keep you going until you have time for something more substantial.

Dried Fruit and Nuts

A handful of unsalted nuts and 6 dried and chopped apricots are a nutrient packed snack that will keep you on the go until the next meal. They're easily portable and unlike some snacks, not in the least bit messy to eat. Put them in a pot or a resealable plastic bag and take wherever you go – you'll never grab snacks full of refined sugar again!

Tip: Nuts are loaded with protein, minerals like zinc, magnesium, and selenium, and antioxidants like vitamin E. They contain fat but it's mostly the beneficial monounsaturated kind. They are also low-GL. However, both apricots and nuts are high in calories so keep to a small amount of each. Try to find organic apricots because they are less likely to have added preservatives.

Nutrient analysis per serving: Calories 261; Protein 9g; Carbohydrate 20g; Fat 16g; Saturated fat 2.5g; Fibre 5g; Sodium 97mg.

Crudités

Take a bag of crudités with you – carrots, cauliflower, celery, apple, broccoli, peppers, and so on – chopped into slices or batons and sealed in a plastic bag to keep them fresh and crunchy.

Tip: Pop them in the fridge where possible, and don't worry if the apple turns a bit brown, it won't harm you.

Nutrient analysis per serving: Calories 40; Protein 0g; Carbohydrate 7g; Fat 0g; Saturated fat 0g; Fibre 2g; Sodium 25mg.

Toasted Seeds

Toasted seeds are a miracle food – throw a handful of your favourite seeds such as sunflower seeds, pumpkin seeds, pine nuts, and so on – into a pan, dry toast them, and let them cool, then throw them into a bag and tie in a knot.

Nutrient analysis per handful: Calories 165; Protein 5g; Carbohydrate 3g; Fat 15g; Saturated fat 1.5g; Fibre 2 grams, 10 milligrams sodium.

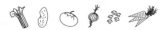

Tucking in to Hot Snacks

Sometimes only a hot tidbit can satisfy a rumbly tum. These recipes are sure to hit the spot and keep you going between meals. Toast is a great comfort food – choose low-GL bread with as many seeds in as you can and top with avocado, sardines, or bean sprouts and cheese.

Avocado Nut Butter on Toast

Avocado makes a great alternative to regular butter or peanut butter. This is a good way to use up ripe fruit rather than making guacamole.

Preparation time: *5 minutes*

Serves: *1*

1 small ripe avocado, stone and scoop flesh out	*1 dash Tabasco or other pepper sauce (optional)*
1 tablespoon fresh lemon juice	*1 tablespoon pine nuts, toasted*
Zest 1 lemon	*2 slices low-GL toast*
Freshly ground black pepper	

Roughly mash the avocado in a bowl with the lemon juice, zest, black pepper, and Tabasco. Stir in the toasted pine nuts. Spread onto hot low-GL toast – yum!

Variation: *Toast pumpkin or sunflower seeds in place of pine nuts; serve with a couple of oatcakes.*

Nutrient analysis per serving: *Calories 338; Protein 6g; Carbohydrate 15g; Fat 28g; Saturated fat 5g; Fibre 5g; Sodium 171mg.*

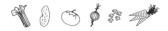

Bean Sprout and Cheese Melt

The bean sprouts add a surprising, nutritious crunch to this old favorite.

Preparation time: *5 minutes*

Serves: *1*

1 teaspoon extra-virgin olive oil

1 dash Tabasco or other pepper sauce (optional)

Handful of bean sprouts

2 slices reduced-fat cheddar cheese – enough to cover the bean sprouts

1 slice low-GL toast

Freshly ground black pepper

1 Preheat your grill (broiler) on the highest setting.

2 Mix the olive oil and Tabasco together (or use an olive oil infused with chilli).

3 Put the sprouts on the toast, and drizzle over the olive oil and Tabasco mix. Scatter over the cheese so that the sprouts are completely covered. Grind over some black pepper, and pop under the grill (broiler) until the cheese is *just* melting. Serve immediately.

Tip: *Spread the toast with avocado nut butter first (see Avocado Nut Butter recipe earlier in this chapter).*

Nutrient analysis per serving: *Calories 185; Protein 14g; Carbohydrate 14g; Fat 8g; Saturated fat 3g; Fibre 2.5g; Sodium 369mg.*

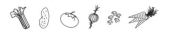

Sardines on Toast

Sometimes the old recipes are the best! Okay, we know this dish isn't exactly original, but take a trip down memory lane by snacking on this tried-and-tested reliable favourite.

Preparation and cooking time: *7 minutes*

Serves: *1*

1 tin (100g) sardines in olive oil, drained

1 teaspoon Worcestershire sauce

1 slice low-GL toast

30 grams / 1 ounce / 2 tablespoons reduced-fat mature cheddar, coarsely grated

1 Preheat the grill (broiler) to very hot.

2 Mash the sardines up in a bowl with the Worcester sauce. Spread the mixture on the toast, top with the cheese, and grill until melted. Grind over some fresh black pepper – delicious!

Nutrient analysis per serving: Calories 360; Protein 36g; Carbohydrate 13g; Fat 19g; Saturated fat 6g; Fibre 1.5g; Sodium 1073mg.

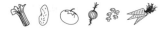

Baked Veggie Skewers

These easy and delicious vegetable skewers are perfect with a couple of slices of scrummy hard cheese such as Manchego (a type of ewe's cheese from Spain), or rounds of soft goat's cheese.

Preparation time: *5 minutes*

Cooking time: *40 minutes*

Serves: *Makes 6 skewers*

2 courgettes (zucchini), cut into 1-inch chunks

1 aubergine (eggplant), cut into 1-inch chunks

Half a sweet potato, peeled and cut into ½-inch chunks

2 tablespoons extra-virgin olive oil

1 tablespoon balsamic vinegar

1 garlic clove, crushed or grated

Freshly ground black pepper

1 In a bowl, mix the vegetable chunks with the oil, vinegar, and garlic.

2 Thread the vegetables onto small skewers (soak wooden skewers in water first to prevent them from burning), and arrange on a baking tray with plenty of room between each skewer.

3 Pop into a medium oven (350°F / 180°C / Gas Mark 4) to cook for about 35 to 40 minutes until soft.

Nutrient analysis per stick: Calories 56; Protein 1g; Carbohydrate 4g; Fat 4g; Saturated fat 0.5g; Fibre 1.5g; Sodium 7mg.

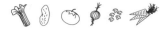

Peach and Bacon Grill'ems

This little tempter is an example of how sweet and savoury can be a real hit when you bring them together. Delicious!

Preparation time: *4 minutes*

Cooking time: *6 minutes*

1 ripe peach, cut into quarters

2 rashers (strips) smoked lean bacon, cut in half

1 Wrap each peach quarter in half a rasher of smoked bacon, and push through a cocktail stick to secure (soak wooden sticks in water so they don't burn).

2 Cook in a frying pan or skillet over a medium heat for 4–6 minutes, turning several times until the bacon is cooked and the peach becomes soft and starts to release its juices. Serve immediately.

Variation: *Replace the peach with strawberries (halved or whole depending on their size) or thick slices of fresh apricot.*

Nutrient analysis per canapé: Calories 71; Protein 6g; Carbohydrate 3g; Fat 4g; Saturated fat 1.5g; Fibre 0.5g; Sodium 448mg.

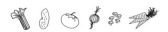

Part IV
Optimising GL

The 5th Wave   By Rich Tennant

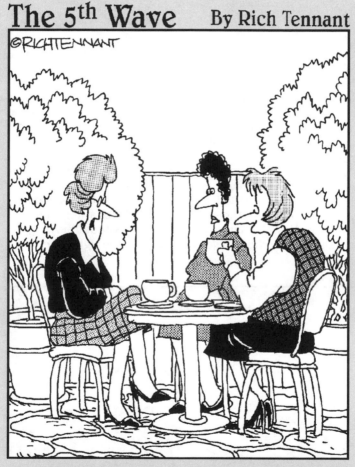

"Oh, I have a very healthy relationship with food. It's the relationship I have with my scale that's not so good."

In this part . . .

*P*art IV gives you all the know-how to make popular recipes GL-friendly. We also explain how the other parts of the healthy eating jigsaw fit into the low-GL eating plan so that the GL Diet can be a way of life rather than a quick fix. You find out how to get active without blowing a gasket and also how to get your head in the right place for success.

Chapter 11

Replacing Common Ingredients with GL-friendly Alternatives

*O*ne of the key features of any successful diet for weight loss, or any other specific aim for that matter, is that the diet has to be flexible. Lists of banned foods and rigid rules simply don't work. The trouble with rules and regulations is that at some point, either wittingly or by accident, you find yourself in a situation when you break the rules. When you're following a diet, breaking the rules often leads to shattered confidence, lost resolve, and that horrible cycle of yo-yo dieting.

The good news is that you won't find any rigid rules and regulations in this book, just helpful and practical guidelines and tips to help you make the right choices for a healthy, happy, low-GL way of life.

We want to equip you so well that you naturally choose a low-GL alternative to a high-GL food choice. This chapter guides you through some easy tips for making the best low-GL choices when your options are limited. We also give you some general pointers to help you make traditional favourite foods and recipes more GL friendly and best of all, we tell you everything you need to know to keep your GL diet as flexible as possible.

Breaking Your Potato Habit

Don't get us wrong, we're not anti-potatoes! However, the structure of a potato and some of the ways you cook them make potatoes high-GL. Large white potatoes, boiled to a pulp, is a recipe for GL disaster. Follow our tips to help you keep potatoes, and some great alternatives, on the menu.

Smashing mashing

A steaming bowl of smooth, creamy mashed potatoes is surely one of the most comforting foods in the world. Usually, you use large white flowery potatoes to make mashed potato, which is not great news for your GL and stablising your blood sugars.

But don't write off mashed potato for good. You can make a great chunky potato crush with baby new potatoes. Keep the skins on the potatoes and boil until cooked, then crush them with a fork so that the potatoes are just broken rather than smooth. Add a little butter or low-fat spread and some black pepper. Alternatively, add some natural yoghurt and fresh chopped chives – delicious.

A whole host of other veggies make great tasting, colourful mash. You can use them for topping on dishes such as fish pie or shepherd's pie, or simply use mash as a side vegetable.

The basic recipe is to peel, chop, boil the vegetables in water until cooked, and then, you guessed it, mash! (See? You're a great cook after all!)

Great alternative mash combos include:

- ✔ **Cauli mash:** Try this dish before you say a thing! Boil a whole cauliflower, then mash with a little mustard, some crème fraîche, and black pepper. This combination is the creamiest mash you'll ever eat!

- ✔ **Celeriac and herb mash:** The poor celeriac is probably one of the ugliest veggies you'll ever see, but get past the peeling and simply treat it like mashed potatoes. Add parsley or basil. This slightly aniseed flavoured mash goes brilliantly with rich sauces and gravies.

✔ **Carrot and swede mash:** Two vibrant looking and tasting veggies that were just meant to be together.

✔ **Carrot and sweet potato mash:** This mash is great for children – bright orange with just a touch of sweetness.

Coasting for a roasting

The Sunday roast is often one of the few times in a week when the whole family comes together for a meal. We don't want to leave you thinking that you can't have your weekend treat with your nearest and dearest.

Simply follow these top tips for keeping the GL lid on your roast:

✔ Choose leaner cuts of meat and poultry.

✔ Instead of roast potatoes, roast a selection of the following vegetables for a change: carrots, sweet potatoes, celeriac, butternut squash, and red onions.

✔ Serve plenty of steamed vegetables, and aim for three or four different side dishes of vegetables.

✔ Use a teaspoon of cornflour to thicken gravy, and skim off any excess fat from meat juices.

Sweet potatoes also make great baked potatoes. You can cook them in the oven or the microwave and they're delicious with cottage cheese and chives.

If I'd Known You Were Coming, I'd Have Baked a Cake!

Bet you didn't think you'd find tips for baking cakes in a book with 'diet' in the title! We love food too much to ban anything. Admittedly, if you're trying to lose weight a slice of cake every day is not such a great idea, but remember – the GL Diet is a diet for life, not just a week or so. Now, at some time in your long and healthy life you're sure to have a birthday, or Christmas, right? A special occasion calls for a cake, and we can share a few simple tips to lower the GL of your cakes and desserts.

The main ingredients that you're looking to replace in a cake recipe are the sugar and the white flour. You can make a fantastic sponge cake using equal quantities of 100 per cent wholemeal flour and almond flour. Use fructose instead of sugar but remember that you only need two-thirds of the amount in the recipe because fructose tastes much sweeter than table sugar.

Fructose browns more quickly at high temperatures than regular sugar, so slightly reduce the recommended oven temperature and keep an eye on your cake while cooking.

If you want to make your sponge extra special, swap sugar-filled icing, frosting, or jam for delicious fresh fruit such as strawberries and a dash of low-fat crème fraîche.

Rumble for a crumble

Fruit crumbles are a real traditional, old fashioned pudding. Show us a person who doesn't like crumble and we'll eat our . . . crumble! The fruit is good for you, but the traditional crumble topping is full of flour and sugar – not helpful when you're trying to eat low GL.

Here's our tried and tested low-GL crumble topping, which our friends and families love:

225 grams / 8 ounces / 1 cup old fashioned porridge oats

1 teaspoon ground cinnamon

50 grams / 1½ ounces / ¼ cup ground almonds

2 tablespoons fructose (fruit sugar)

1 tablespoon butter or olive oil spread

1 Put all the ingredients in a bowl and rub together with your fingertips until you have a crumbly mixture.

2 Then add the crumble to your favourite softened fruit. Apple and blackberry, apple and pear, rhubarb, raspberries, blackcurrants, and gooseberries all work brilliantly in a crumble. Soften the fruit by gently heating it in a pan with a little water for a few minutes.

3 Simply bake in a hot oven for 20 to 30 minutes or until golden brown. Serve with low-fat crème fraîche or natural yoghurt.

Cheeky cheesecakes

Cheesecake isn't exactly the best dessert to choose when you're trying to lose weight. However, for the odd special occasion you can make this dish as a low-GL dessert by reducing the amount of sugar and using lots of different fresh fruit in the topping. For the sweet biscuit base try using ground nuts such as almonds with a tablespoon of fructose and a little butter or olive oil spread instead of smashed digestive biscuits. Plain low-fat cream cheese topped with fresh fruit makes a great topping.

Cheesecake is still a calorie-packed pud, so cut yourself a small portion.

Flour Power: Choosing Low-GL Alternatives

You can easily make a lot of recipes healthier by reducing the amount of sugar, salt, or fat in the standard recipe. Perhaps you are used to doing that routinely. When a recipe calls for flour, omitting the flour is a bit trickier: sauces don't thicken, cakes don't rise, and breads simply don't work!

We've experimented with all sorts of different flours to save you time and frustration. We can't promise that you won't have one or two disappointments, but we can give you tips on which flours work best in certain recipes. All the flours we mention have a lower GL than regular white flour.

Using your loaf

People are often given a breadmaker as a gift – one they never use. Breadmakers seem like a good idea at the time, but all too often they live out their days in the back of a kitchen cupboard.

Your time has come to take up the challenge and start baking! Homemade bread is so easy to make, and fills the house with the most irresistible aroma. You can exchange high-GL flours for spelt or rye flour, which have a much lower GL and give a lovely nutty flavour to bread.

The main rule with bread recipe adaptation is to make sure that the low-GL dry ingredients all add up to the total dry ingredients in the original recipe. You can use oats, oatbran, and rye flakes to replace some of the flour, but you also need to mix in a quantity of rye or spelt flour.

Replacing white flour means that your end product is not quite as light and fluffy as usual, but don't give up, and keep experimenting.

Adding a few tablespoons of seeds such as flaxseeds, linseeds, or sesame seeds and some crushed nuts also lowers the GL and gives the bread a great moist texture. Bread with bits in always has a lower GL than bread without.

Enough of your sauce!

Although the amount of flour you need to thicken a sauce is small, small changes all add up to make a big difference. Check out the following alternative low-GL thickeners, all of which work well.

- ✔ Gram flour and nut flours are good in savoury sauces, and a small amount of cornflour is fine to thicken gravy.

- ✔ Alternatively, you can have a traditional jus (the meat juices), rather than a thickened gravy.

- ✔ Use xanthum gum and ground arrowroot to thicken clear sauces. Both are readily available in supermarkets.

Flipping mad for pancakes and crepes

Buckwheat has a lower GL than regular flour and makes really tasty pancakes. Simply replace the total amount of flour in a pancake recipe with buckwheat for a real American favourite – but then don't ruin all that clever recipe adaptation with lashings of maple syrup! Some fresh lemon juice and a little fructose is a good alternative topping.

Controlling Portion Sizes

We give you all the tips you need for eating out in different restaurants in Chapter 5; in this section we want to save you having arguments or upsetting a gracious host who's spent all day slaving over a stove to prepare a fabulous dinner for you. The last thing you want to do when you receive an invitation to lunch or dinner is call ahead with a whole list of dietary requests. At best your host will think you're a bit of a bore, and at worst he or she will never ask you for dinner again!

Sometimes, saying nothing is the best policy. Don't be overly worried if the meal doesn't tick all the low-GL principles. (Check out the 80/20 Rule in Chapter 12.)

A trick for limiting the damage is to fill your plate the GL-friendly way.

Imagine dividing your plate into quarters. Now fill two quarters with vegetables, one quarter with protein, and one quarter with carbs. Figure 11-1 shows you how. Simply remember 'veggie veggie protein carbs'.

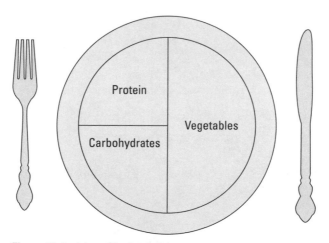

Figure 11-1: A low-GL plateful!

Another way to limit the damage from a less than GL-friendly meal is to reduce the total amount of food you eat. This tip sounds obvious, but you can find exercising portion caution difficult without looking as if you're trying to guess the weight of foods. Try to always serve yourself, rather than allowing your generous host to pile food on your plate.

To judge the overall size of your meal, estimate whether you could fit all the food on your plate into your cupped hands. Have a look at your cupped hands now. Yippee for those of you with big hands!

Your cupped hands represent your stomach. This method is a rough guide but will help you avoid indulging in large quantities of high-GL foods.

Chapter 12

Placing GL in the Healthy Living Jigsaw

In This Chapter
▶ Recognising the importance of a healthy body weight
▶ Understanding and using energy balance to your advantage
▶ Appreciating the benefits of physical activity
▶ Enjoying eating the foods you love – guilt-free

*T*he low-GL way of eating is really healthy, but your diet is only one part of the jigsaw that makes up a healthy lifestyle. In this chapter, we take a look at the other pieces of the puzzle to see how you can fit them together with your low-GL plan to achieve optimum health.

This chapter explains the vital balance between your energy (calorie) intake and your energy expenditure. You can also find out what your ideal healthy weight really is.

Food isn't simply an entry on a 'calories in' balance sheet! Eating is a pleasurable experience with many benefits other than physical health alone. We explore the psychological relationship you have with your food and how you can maximise your enjoyment without compromising your health.

Battling the Bulge: Losing Excess Weight

Being overweight or obese affects nearly every part of your body. Overweight people have a higher risk of developing a variety of illnesses, such as type 2 diabetes, heart disease, high blood pressure, and over 20 types of cancers, including cancer of the colon, breast, uterus, prostate, and stomach. Overweight people have an increased risk of liver disease, gout, gall stones, osteoarthritis of the knee and hip joints, back pain, asthma, and even infertility. Overweight people can also suffer from breathlessness, experience difficulties with walking and sleeping, and be affected by low self-esteem and poor body image. Not very happy reading.

We're here to help you banish these risks! In this section, we look at how you can assess your own health risks and explore the benefits you can expect to gain from shedding any excess pounds.

What is a healthy weight, anyway?

Sorry to burst your bubble, but an *ideal* weight doesn't really exist because everyone is unique. However, you can know the healthy weight range for your height. Recent studies show that as many as one in three men and one in ten women who are overweight believe that they are a healthy weight. You can use our guidelines to accurately assess whether you're within the healthy weight range.

Great big Britain

The number of people who are overweight or obese is rapidly increasing in the United Kingdom. The latest National Diet and Nutrition Survey shows that 25 per cent of men and 20 per cent of women are obese. A further 42 per cent of men and 32 per cent of women are overweight. If this trend continues, nearly half of the British population will be obese by the year 2010. Even more worrying is the marked increase in obesity amongst children. Around one in five British children are now overweight, and one in ten are obese.

The cost to the National Health Service in treating obesity is about £485 million a year, and obesity-related problems result in 18 million sick days a year.

Calculating your Body Mass Index

The *Body Mass Index (BMI)* is a number that measures the relationship between your weight and height and offers an estimate of your risk of weight-related disease.

To calculate your BMI, measure your height in metres (take your shoes off) and your weight in kilograms (definitely take your shoes off!). Now multiply the figure for your height by itself (square it). Divide your weight (in kilograms) by your height (in metres) squared.

BMI = weight (kilograms) / height (metres) × height (metres)

For example, if you are 1.6 metres (5'3") tall and weigh 70 kilograms (11 stone) the equations for your BMI look like this:

$$\text{BMI} = \frac{70}{1.6 \times 1.6} = \frac{70}{2.6} = 27$$

Now you can use Table 12-1 to see how your BMI relates to your weight.

Table 12-1   Classification of Weight Categories Using BMI

BMI	Category
Less than 18.5	Underweight. You may need to gain weight.
18.5–24.9	Normal weight. Aim to stay that way.
25–29.9	Overweight (grade 1 obesity). Weight loss may help your health. Avoid further weight gain.
30–39.9	Obese (grade 2 obesity). Your health is at risk. Losing weight will improve your health.
More than 40	Morbid obesity (grade 3 obesity). Visit your doctor for specialist help to manage your weight loss.

Information from World Health Organisation (1997)

Current nutritional research suggests that the healthiest BMI is around 21.0. A BMI higher than 28 doubles your risk of illness and weight-related death.

In Table 12-1, you can see a range of BMIs is given for each category. If you have a small frame with proportionately more fat tissue than muscle tissue (muscle is heavier than fat), you're probably at the low end of the range. If you have a large frame with proportionately more muscle than fat, you're likely to be at the high end.

BMI is not a perfect method for determining your weight because the calculation doesn't measure your body fat specifically; BMI takes into account your *total* weight rather than just fat. If BMI is the only measure used to calculate ideal weight, very muscular people can be mistakenly classified as overweight or even obese. So, what would be a good additional measure? Evidence from population studies suggests that *central obesity* is a serious health risk. Central obesity is where excess weight is stored mainly around your middle or abdomen – the 'apple shape', rather than around the hips and bottom, the 'pear shape'.

Excess fat within the abdominal cavity, which is reflected in an apple shape, causes problems in your body, such as resistance to levels of circulating insulin, increasing blood fats, and the production of cancer-causing agents.

Measuring your waist circumference

Measuring your waist circumference, to assess your level of abdominal fat, or central obesity, is another guide to determining whether your health is at risk. You can measure your waist circumference with a simple tape measure but you must do so in the right place. Pass the tape around your waist level with the upper edge of your hipbone whilst breathing out gently. The tape should fit flat and snug to the skin but not compress it.

Table 12-2 shows the health risk classifications based on waist circumference measurements. South Asian men are especially at risk from central obesity so the cut-off point for 'increased risk' starts at a lower waist circumference.

Measuring waist circumference is also a useful way to monitor the effects of any healthy eating plan or weight-loss diet – a reduction of one centimetre is equal to approximately one kilogram of body fat loss.

Table 12-2	Waist Circumference Classifications		
	Healthy Level	*Level 1: Increased health risk*	*Level 2: Substantially increased health risk*
Men	Less than 94 cm (37 in)	More than 94 cm (37 in)	More than 102 cm (40 in)
South Asian Men	Less than 90 cm (36 in)	More than 90 cm (36 in)	
Women	Less than 80 cm (32 in)	More than 80 cm (32 in)	More than 88 cm (35 in)

World Health Organisation, 1998

Recently researchers have come up with an even easier way to assess health risk. Not surprisingly, your waist circumference is reflected in your clothing size. However, clothing manufacturers measure waist size at a slightly narrower point. Increased health risk is equivalent to a trouser waist size of 34 inches for men and a UK dress size 14 for women. Substantially increased risk is equivalent to above a 36-inch trouser waist for men and a UK dress size 16 for women.

Health benefits of losing weight

If you're overweight, you only need to lose around 5 to 10 per cent of your body weight to gain important health benefits. A person weighing 100 kilograms (15½ stone) can significantly benefit from losing just six kilograms (12 pounds). Based on a loss rate of half a kilogram (1 pound) per week, that's only going to take 3 months! If you lose this amount of weight you're likely to have more energy and feel better before you even start to notice any other physical health benefits.

The health benefits arising from a 10 per cent body weight loss if you're overweight or obese are:

- ✔ Up to 40 per cent reduction in diabetes-related death
- ✔ Half the chance of death from an obesity-related cancer such as breast or colon cancer
- ✔ A substantial reduction in high blood pressure
- ✔ A 10–15 per cent drop in cholesterol levels
- ✔ A rise in good cholesterol levels
- ✔ Up to half the risk of developing type 2 diabetes or high blood sugar levels

Tipping the Energy Balance in Your Favour

Whether you need to lose body fat or simply avoid adding on any more weight, understanding the concept of *energy balance* is crucial. The fat or energy stored in your body is made from any excess you take in from food or drink that you don't use. *Excess* is any food energy or calories over and above what you burn up each day from physical activity and keeping your body in working order. In a nutshell, if you eat roughly the same number of calories as you burn up each day, you keep your weight reasonably steady. If you consistently eat more than you use up, you save the excess in your body bank as fat, with the intention of spending it at a later date! At the other end of the spectrum, if you consistently burn up more energy (calories) than you take in, you start to lose fat stores.

Happily, the GL Diet doesn't involve monitoring the calorie content of every mouthful, or painfully watching the amount calories you burn up on the treadmill. However, GL doesn't ignore energy balance altogether.

Getting energy from food

Energy intake or calories (kcals) comes from food and drink. All foods contain some calories – yes, even celery! The number of calories varies according to the nutritional makeup of the food. Different nutrients provide different amounts of energy per gram, as we show in Table 12-3.

Table 12-3	Energy Content of Main Nutrients
Nutrient	*Energy (calories per gram)*
Fat	9
Carbohydrate	3.75
Protein	4
Alcohol	7

Table 12-3 shows that fat has more calories than carbohydrates. Weight for weight, high-fat foods such as butter or margarine have more energy, or calories, than high-protein or high-carbohydrate foods such as rump steak or bread. You can see that alcohol, which is high in sugar and therefore high-carbohydrate, has a high calorific value. Most fruit and vegetables have a high water content and are low-carbohydrate, so contain less calories.

Every half a kilogram (1 pound) of body fat is equivalent to 3,500 calories of stored energy. If you reduce your energy intake by just 500 calories (2 and a half pints of beer or half a deep pan pizza) a day you can lose 0.5 kilograms (1 pound) of fat a week, or 2 kilograms (4 pounds) per month. If you are overweight, losing five to ten per cent of your body weight (see the section 'Health benefits of losing weight' earlier in this chapter) is easily achievable.

Eating the low-GL way to control energy intake

Eating the low-GL way helps you to feel less hungry by controlling your blood sugar and insulin levels, which means that you can be more successful at cutting down on that 500 calories a day. The GL Diet is enjoyable and easy, so you can follow it for the long term, and, combined with increased physical activity, is the best way to control your weight, permanently!

A growing number of scientific and medical studies are proving that the low glycaemic approach is a safe and sound option for people who need to lose weight.

Large population studies in the United States show that individuals who eat a low-GL diet with less carbohydrate from sugar and refined starches and more from wholegrains, fruit, and vegetables tend to maintain a lower body weight than people not eating low-GL foods.

Recent dietary trials suggest that rather than low-*fat* diets, the most successful weight-loss diet is a nutritionally balanced *energy* restricted diet where both the total amount and the type of carbohydrate are considered – the GL Diet.

Low-glyacemic foods release their sugar into your bloodstream more slowly than high-glycaemic foods, which helps to curb your hunger and leads you to achieve weight loss.

But that's not all. A low-GL diet seems to decrease circulating insulin levels, which in turn decreases your appetite. A study in the United Kingdom shows that people who eat a low-GL breakfast experience significantly reduced feelings of hunger throughout the day. Those eating a high-GL breakfast were hungrier by lunchtime. Furthermore, low-GL breakfast eaters actually ate *less* than usual at lunch later that day. Eating the low-GL way makes you feel less tired, less cold, and less hungry – which all trigger eating – and more likely to stick to the diet in the long term. Head to Chapter 6 for our low-GL breakfasts.

Choose low-GL foods at meals and snack times to stop the peaks and troughs in your blood sugar and insulin that make you feel hungry. If you experience fewer cravings for high calorie, high-fat, high-sugar foods, your overall calorie or energy intake will reduce. Head to Chapter 10 for our low-GL snacks to help you beat the mid-morning munchies.

On Your Bike, Mate: Getting Active

Okay, so you can tip the energy balance in your favour by controlling your food intake. The other side of the scales is your energy *expenditure* or output.

Even when you think that you're resting, your body is busy burning up energy. Your heart beats. Your lungs expand and contract. Your intestines digest food. Your muscles work gently. Cells send electrical impulses, and your brain continually signals to every part of your body.

The energy that your resting body uses is called (quite appropriately) *resting energy expenditure,* and accounts for a massive 60 to 70 per cent of the total calories you need each day. The other 30 to 40 per cent comes from the physical exercise you do each day. Just like a car, moving muscles need fuel and they take what they need from your energy stores. You can use physical activity to tip the energy balance even more in your favour.

When you engage in physical activity you don't just burn calories during the activity but also for some time afterwards. Contrary to popular belief, working out doesn't make you feel hungrier – in fact, physical activity works with your low-GL diet plan to make controlling your appetite easier. Being active helps to increase the proportion of fat lost in relation to muscle, and helps you to maintain your weight loss.

Reaping the rewards

Physical activity has many other health benefits over and above weight control, making exercise an important piece of the healthy lifestyle jigsaw. Irrespective of weight, physical activity helps to reduce the risk of coronary heart disease by lowering *LDL cholesterol* (the type of circulating fat that can block the blood vessels) and promoting good HDL cholesterol that protects against blocked blood vessels.

Several studies in the United States and Finland show that physical activity combined with a healthy diet can help prevent type 2 diabetes by up to 58 per cent in high risk groups (see Chapter 13 for more on coronary heart disease and diabetes). Physical activity also helps reduce high blood pressure levels and prevents the natural tendency for the pressure to rise as we get older. Regular weight-bearing activity helps to keep your bones strong, protecting against osteoporosis.

The benefits of getting active aren't simply physical. Exercise can also build self-esteem and stimulates the production of those feel-good hormones or *endorphins*, natural highs that improve your mood, help prevent depression and anxiety, enable you to cope with stress, and make you sleep better.

Small increases in activity can lead to noticeable health gains no matter how old or how fit you are when you start, and you don't have to be a top-notch athlete to reap the benefits.

On your marks

Check with your doctor before starting to exercise if you haven't been active for a while or have any medical problems. Your doctor can advise you about the best type and level of exercise for you. Whatever exercise you do, start slowly and build up gradually, increasing the intensity and length of sessions as you get fitter. Don't do too much too soon or you can hurt yourself!

Choose an activity that you enjoy, can afford to do, and can fit into your lifestyle to ensure that you stick with it. You may find exercising with a friend motivational. Physical activity doesn't have to be competitive sport or gym-based workouts although you may find these forms of exercise very motivating. Activities that are brisk or of *moderate intensity* and use fat as an energy source seem to be the most beneficial to health. 'Brisk' means just enough to get you a little hot and sweaty, and to speed up your breathing, heartbeat, and pulse rate without you becoming uncomfortably out of breath – slightly breathless, but not speechless!

Moderate-intensity activities include:

- ✔ Brisk walking
- ✔ Dancing
- ✔ Cycling
- ✔ Gym classes, such as low-impact aerobics, martial arts, and spinning (indoor cycling on a stationary bike set to music)
- ✔ Jogging or running

✔ Swimming or water aerobics

✔ Team sports, such as football, rugby, and hockey

✔ Tennis

Some GPs can provide 'exercise on prescription' to patients with heart disease risk factors such as high blood pressure, diabetes, obesity, or high cholesterol. These may include vouchers for swimming, exercise classes, or a course of gym sessions at your local leisure centre.

Resistance training, using light weights, builds muscle strength and flexibility. Make sure that you warm up your body beforehand and cool it down afterwards.

Drink plenty of water before, during, and after activity. You sweat to cool yourself down and so you need to replace the water you lose to prevent yourself from overheating.

Walking to keep fit

Brisk walking is a great form of exercise – and it's free! To get a real health benefit and improvement in fitness you need to be walking briskly for 30 minutes or more at least five days a week. If you want to lose weight, then 45 to 60 minutes is optimal.

Don't panic at the time periods involved – you don't have to do the walking all in one go. Bite-sized chunks of 10 to 15 minutes spread throughout the day are just as effective.

You can wear a *pedometer*, or step counter, on your belt to monitor the number of steps you take each day and to give you a good measure of how much activity you do. Simple, inexpensive models are available in sports shops and chemists. Two thousand steps equates to about one kilometre. A recent study in the United States shows that asking people to build up to 10,000 steps a day is more effective and motivational than asking people to walk for 30 minutes a day. Check your daily average over a week and see if you need to be walking more. Table 12-4 gives you the step counts equivalent of different activity levels. Aim to be active, with 10,000 steps a day.

Table 12-4 Steps per Day for Different Activity Levels	
Steps per day	*Activity level*
Under 5,000	Sedentary
5,000–7,499	Average
7,500–9,999	Above average
Over 10,000	Active
Over 12,500	Highly active

Being physically active is fun, sociable, gives you goals to aim for and a sense of achievement – so what are you waiting for?

Enjoying Your Food: More Pleasure and Less Guilt

As registered dietitians, we look at food as a way of providing nutrients for health. However, even we poor nutritionists know that eating is more than about just that! We are both real foodies and get great satisfaction from eating and drinking. Cooking meals and sharing them with friends and family also play an important social role in our lives. The final piece of our healthy lifestyle jigsaw puzzle is about promoting an enjoyable and healthy relationship with food.

Humans are genetically designed to enjoy foods that we know are safe and familiar to us. Studies show that when we smell, taste, or even simply catch sight of our favourite foods, endorphins, which regulate feelings of pleasure and mood, are released into our brain.

We're always saddened when people, for whatever reason, deny themselves this satisfaction by banning their favourite foods and then feeling guilty when they give in to temptation. Part of the appeal of the low-GL way of eating is that no food is forbidden. No healthy eating plan should make you feel bad about what you eat, insist that you eat certain foods or particular combinations of foods with magical properties, or suggest that you cut out entire food groups.

Good and bad foods or good and bad diets?

'Good' and 'bad' foods don't exist, only 'good' and 'bad' diets. However, some foods are designed to play centre stage in your diet (think fruit and vegetables and low-GL carbs). Other foods are more suited for the walk-on parts and smaller roles (think high-fat, high-sugar foods with few other nutrients). Take cream for instance. Cream is low in GL but high in saturated fat and calories. If you load your coffee or drown your dessert with cream you're overdoing it. However, a tablespoon of cream on a bowl of fruit transforms it into a delicious dessert. So we use small amounts in some of our dessert recipes in Chapter 9. Yum!

Following the 80/20 Rule

No one is perfect 100 per cent of the time – that would make for a very dull world! The good news is that you don't need to be perfect on the GL Diet.

The 80/20 Rule means that for 80 per cent of the time you choose from a variety of healthy, nutritious foods. The other 20 per cent of the time you relax and choose small portions of your favourite, less nutritious foods that might provide very few other nutrients but lots of pleasure. What could be simpler than having your cake and eating it, but less of it, less often?

Food: An emotional experience

The Lean Habits Study is the world's largest study of successful weight maintenance. This ground-breaking study began in the late 1990s and is looking at the eating habits and lifestyles of 8,000 European participants. The study compares those who are successful at keeping to a healthy weight over several years with those who are less successful and identifies the dietary behaviours that are most effective; the so-called 'lean habits'.

The Lean Habits Study reveals a lot about the importance of how people think and feel about food. An overriding message from the study is the need to be flexible about eating. The study shows that rigid rules and restrictions are destined to failure and the 'all or nothing' way of thinking (either denying yourself a certain food all together, or going completely overboard and overeating it) is particularly unhelpful. For example, in social situations you're better off relaxing a little and choosing a few treat foods rather than eating nothing (= no fun) or thinking 'there's nothing healthy here so I might as well go overboard' (= guilt). So, have a little fun and don't feel guilty – which is good for you!

The study identified several other successful strategies involving thoughts and feelings around food:

- Allow treats of particularly enjoyable foods.

- Have no forbidden foods and plenty of variety and choice.

- Cope with stress, anger, boredom, or sadness in ways other than eating, such as phoning a friend, doing some exercise, having a relaxing bath, solving a puzzle, or reading your favourite magazine.

- Be kind to yourself if you slip up or have a set back in moving towards a healthier way of eating.

If you want to find out more about the complex psychological relationship between people and food, the following sources may be helpful:

- The Obesity Awareness and Solutions Trust (TOAST) www.toast-uk.org.uk, or 0845 045 0225. TOAST is a charity dedicated to providing information, help, and support in the prevention and treatment of obesity.

- The Eating Disorders Association www.edauk.com, or 0845 634 1414. The charity provides help and support to people whose lives have been affected by an eating disorder.

- Overeaters Anonymous www.oa.org, or www.oagb.org.uk. OA is a worldwide registered charity for people who suffer from periods of overeating and obsession with weight or food issues.

Chapter 13

Medical Benefits of the GL Diet

· ·

· ·

*A*dopting a low-GL diet is not just a great eating plan to control your weight. GL focuses on carbohydrate management, but it also embraces all the other aspects of a healthy diet and lifestyle – the GL Diet is much more than simply a weight-loss tool.

In this chapter we take you on a whistle-stop tour through the science and research that reveals how a low-glycaemic diet is beneficial for your health and well-being, improving the overall health of people with specific conditions, and helping to improve symptoms of common conditions.

Looking at GL and Diabetes

Diabetes mellitus, commonly known simply as diabetes, is a condition in which the amount of glucose in your blood is too high or too low because your body can't use glucose properly. Glucose is your body's fuel and you top it up from the food you eat. Insulin is the hormone produced in the pancreas that keeps glucose under control and helps it get to the cells that need the fuel. Insulin works a bit like the thermostat on your central heating system to keep a constant temperature. People with diabetes have problems either producing or using insulin, so they're in danger of having too much or too little glucose in their blood.

Glucose comes from the digestion of carbohydrate foods, such as bread, rice, potatoes, and cereals, and from sugar and sweet foods, as well as from your liver where you make glucose.

Choosing a low-GL diet makes sense for people with diabetes because low-GL foods release sugar into the bloodstream slowly, which in turn helps to control the release of insulin.

The boffins agree with us: A team of scientists from Colorado State University in the United States looked at the increasing prevalence of type 2 diabetes in urban areas of industrialised countries (type 2 diabetes develops more slowly than type 1, and the symptoms are usually less severe). The scientists found that over the past 200 years, consumption of refined cereals and sugars increased at almost exactly the same rate as type 2 diabetes. The team concluded that the increase of sugar in people's diet was clearly linked to increased levels of insulin, and the subsequent increase in developing type 2 diabetes.

Another study of over 40,000 health professionals working with men reports that a high-glycaemic load diet increased the risk of developing type 2 diabetes. Similar findings in women are reported by the American Medical Association, who found that the women who ate more high-GL foods had a greater incidence of diabetes.

Both the European Association for the Study of Diabetes and Diabetes UK, the leading UK charity for people with diabetes, recommend a low-glycaemic, high-fibre diet as a means of maintaining good control of blood sugars and for helping to maintain a healthy weight.

A low-GL diet as part of a healthy lifestyle can help to control your diabetes and reduces your risk of long-term diabetes-related complications.

Even small changes in your diet can make a big difference! Two large scientific reviews show that a low-glycaemic diet has a positive effect on blood sugar control in people who already have diabetes, and that swapping just one high-glycaemic food for a low-glycaemic alternative can also have a beneficial effect.

Check out *Diabetes For Dummies* by Dr Sarah Jarvis and Alan L. Rubin (Wiley) if you want to find out more about living with diabetes.

Low GL and High Blood Pressure

High blood pressure is also known as the silent killer because the condition often goes undetected. *Blood pressure* is the force exerted by blood on the walls of your arteries when your heart beats.

 Although high blood pressure can cause headaches, dizziness, and problems with vision, the majority of people with high blood pressure suffer no symptoms at all. However, high blood pressure causes heart attacks, strokes, and kidney damage, so have your blood pressure checked by your GP or practice nurse every couple of years or so.

Under pressure: Measuring blood pressure

When a doctor measures your blood pressure, two readings are recorded.

The first reading is for the *systolic pressure*, which represents the force of the blood as your heart contracts (beats) to pump blood around your body. The second reading is for the *diastolic pressure,* which records the pressure of your blood flow while your heart is filling with blood again

in preparation for the next *contraction,* or heart beat. Most healthy people should have a blood pressure reading of less than 140/90. The numbers mean *millimeters of mercury,* a standard unit for the measurement of pressure. Risk of heart attack and stroke increases as these numbers increase (particularly diastolic, the second number).

A low-GL diet is unlikely to directly lower blood pressure that is already high. However, people who are overweight and have high blood pressure can expect to see a significant improvement in their blood pressure when they lose as little as five per cent of their body weight.

If you suffer from high blood pressure, one of the most important things you can do is to limit the amount of salt you eat. Studies show that many people with high blood pressure are also 'salt sensitive', and they can better control their blood pressure when they eat less salt. Following these pointers can help you to lower your salt intake:

- Reduce the amount of processed, manufactured food you eat.

- If you really need to add salt to your food, add it either during cooking or at the table, but not both.

- Avoid eating naturally salty foods such as smoked meats, cured meats and fish, and salty snacks.

For more about salt, check out Chapter 3.

Reducing the Risk of Heart Disease with Low-GL

Coronary heart disease (CHD) occurs when your arteries become narrowed by *atherosclerosis*, a build-up of fatty materials within the walls of your arteries. Atherosclerosis causes a restriction in the supply of blood and oxygen to your heart, particularly when you exert yourself and increase the demands of your heart muscle. Your blood also becomes more prone to clotting.

Atherosclerosis can block the delivery of nutrients to the artery walls, causing them to lose their elasticity. This condition may lead to high blood pressure, which also increases the risk of coronary heart disease.

The main symptom of coronary heart disease is *angina*, caused by insufficient oxygen reaching your heart muscle because of a reduction in blood flow. Angina is a feeling of heaviness, tightness, or pain in the middle of your chest that may affect your arms, neck, jaw, face, back, or abdomen.

Unfortunately, for many people, the first indication that they have CHD is the on-set of a heart attack. A heart attack happens when the blood supply to a part of the heart muscle is interrupted or stops, usually because of a blood clot in the coronary artery.

You can minimise the risk of developing CHD with the GL Diet. Evidence from around the world suggests that a low-glycaemic diet may reduce the risk of heart disease in a number of ways. In 1999, the World Health Organisation and the Food and Agriculture Organisation recommended that people in industrialised countries base their diets on low-glycaemic foods in order to prevent coronary heart disease, diabetes, and obesity.

Several studies show that certain blood fats linked to heart disease were lower in groups of people following a low-glycaemic diet, compared with people following a high-glycaemic diet. Some scientists argue that a low-GL diet is naturally rich in fruits and vegetables, which have a protective role in heart disease and the benefit of a low-GL diet has nothing to do with carbohydrates.

Whatever the reason, a low-GL diet has an important role to play in the prevention of heart disease. The GL Diet is an effective measure against heart disease when integrated into a healthy lifestyle:

- ✔ Be active – 30 minutes a day makes all the difference.

- ✔ Be smoke free. From the moment you stop smoking your risk of a heart attack is reduced, and after one smoke-free year the risk is halved.

- ✔ Keep your alcohol consumption within safe limits (refer to Chapter 5 for more on recommended limits). Binge drinking increases your risk of heart attack. Chapter 5 explains safe alcohol intake.

- ✔ Maintain a healthy weight – following the GL Diet and staying active helps take care of that!

The Metabolic Syndrome – The Secret Killer

The *metabolic syndrome* or *syndrome X* is when a number of different cardiovascular risk factors exist in a person at the same time. This combination of risk factors puts a major strain on the cardiovascular system and increases the likelihood of sufferers going on to develop cardiovascular disease, such as angina, strokes, and heart attack as well as diabetes.

In 2002, a review of all the research since 1981 was published in the *Journal of the American Medical Association*. The authors concluded that eating low-glycaemic foods have a valid role to play in the prevention and treatment of the metabolic syndrome and therefore obesity, diabetes, and cardiovascular disease. Identifying and treating people who display some of the features of the metabolic syndrome is likely to be a crucial part of stopping these follow-on types of diseases in their tracks.

Metabolic syndrome and syndrome X are two names for the same set of symptoms or conditions. The syndrome itself is a precursor for heart disease and diabetes. The key is to detect the people with metabolic syndrome early enough to stop them going on to develop heart disease or diabetes.

Diagnosis of the metabolic syndrome requires three or more of the following features. Your doctor can take these measurements.

- ✔ Abdominal obesity: Waist larger than 102 centimetres (men) or 88 centimetres (women)

- ✔ Fasting blood glucose greater than or equal to 6.1 mmol/l

- ✔ Blood pressure greater than or equal to 130mm Hg (systolic) and/or 85 mm Hg (diastolic)

- ✔ Fasting triglycerides (fats in the blood) greater than 1.71 mmol/L

- ✔ HDL (good) cholesterol less than 1.0 mmol/L (men) or 1.3 mmol/L (women)

Making diet and lifestyle changes can improve these measurements.

Sometimes It's Hard to Be a Woman: Female Health and the GL Diet

A low-GL diet helps to control the release of the hormone insulin. As with diabetics (refer to the 'Looking at GL and Diabetes' section earlier in this chapter), many women find a low-GL diet helps to improve hormonally driven symptoms associated with pre-menstrual syndrome, polycystic ovary syndrome, and the menopause.

The GL Diet can really help if you suffer from symptoms induced by hormonal change such as *pre-menstrual syndrome* and *polycystic ovary syndrome*. However, don't expect overnight results. From our experience, women usually feel improvements in their symptoms up to three months after a change in their diet. So, stick to the GL Diet and monitor the reduction of your symptoms.

Pre-menstrual syndrome (PMS)

Pre-menstrual syndrome (PMS) is the name given to the disruptive physiological symptoms that appear regularly before a period, but improve when bleeding begins. PMS is a serious medical condition that affects one in three women. PMS is often worse at either end of your reproductive life: around *puberty* and before the *menopause*. PMS can be more of a problem after childbirth, during your 30s and 40s, and during times of stress.

More than 150 symptoms are associated with PMS. A woman's individual symptoms can vary from month to month and can appear up to two weeks before a period.

The most common symptoms include:

- Depression and agitation
- Breast tenderness
- Fluid retention and *bloating*
- Irritability and mood swings
- Headaches
- Skin and hair changes

Polycystic ovary syndrome (PCOS)

Polycystic ovary syndrome (PCOS) affects up to ten per cent of women, although many don't realise that they're suffering from the condition.

Typical symptoms include:

- Pain from cysts on the ovaries
- Infertility
- High blood pressure
- Acne
- Central obesity (putting on weight around your middle)
- Baldness or, conversely, excessive body hair
- Irregular periods

Scientists don't know the cause of PCOS. However, new research suggests that PCOS may be linked to raised levels of insulin, which stimulate the ovaries to produce too much testosterone. Your body becomes resistant to the effects of insulin, so your pancreas produces higher and higher levels of insulin to get the same effect. Insulin is produced in response to glucose in the blood from food. Peaks of blood sugar from a high-GL diet cause insulin to work even harder in someone with PCOS. Many dietitians working with patients suffering from PCOS recommend a low-GL diet to help control this double-whammy insulin effect.

 For more information and advice on PCOS, head to www. verity-pcos.org.uk. See your GP for the many different treatments available for PCOS.

The menopause

The *menopause* is the time when a woman's fertility winds down. The menopause doesn't need to mean new restrictions or physical decline; many women find that the menopause opens new opportunities to them and is a very positive time of their life. Menopause starts to occur in most women around their 50th year, although this can vary. Some women face the menopause much earlier or later than this.

As you go through the menopause, your ovaries produce less of the hormone oestrogen. This reduction triggers the brain to release other hormones in an attempt to make the ovaries work harder. The number and quality of eggs released – and thus fertility – decreases.

Symptoms such as hot flushes, sweats, muscle and bone pains, irritability, and poor concentration are all linked to these hormonal surges.

The GL Diet can be beneficial to menopausal women in a number of ways:

- ✔ Menopausal symptoms are hormone related, and the GL Diet improves the control of the hormone insulin.

- ✔ Stable blood sugars improve poor concentration and irritability.

- ✔ Many menopausal women find that they gradually gain weight. The GL Diet is effective at helping to control weight.

- ✔ The menopause is a time when a woman's risk of heart disease increases, and the GL Diet protects against heart disease.

Hey, Wake Up at the Back!

Most people experience lapses in concentration when you lose your trail of thought or drift off into your imagination for a few brief moments. Don't worry – that is quite normal! Often, people can really struggle to stay awake, let alone concentrate, at specific times of the day, typically mid morning and mid afternoon, and this can be a problem when you're at work or school.

Your brain uses glucose in preference to the other organs in the body that need glucose – in short, if the brain doesn't get fuel then everything else slows down, and that's when you get sleepy.

Studies in the UK show that children who eat a breakfast cereal in the morning perform better and are better able to concentrate. Choosing a low-GL breakfast such as porridge or an oat-based cereal, and eating low-GL meals and snacks throughout the day have a similar effect in contributing to this improved performance.

Eating the low-GL way means that you give your body a steady drip-feed of energy so that you can keep going for longer.

Part V
The Part of Tens

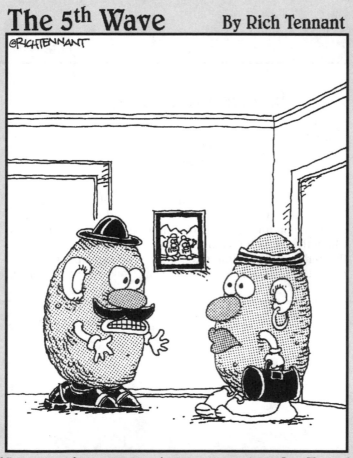

"Look, you're never going to look like Mrs. French Fry, or Mrs. Cheese Stick. Besides, do you have any idea what their cholesterol levels are?"

In this part . . .

No *For Dummies* book is complete without the Part of Tens. We've packed this part full with nifty lists of essential GL-related information that you can access quickly and easily.

Discover great reasons for choosing low-GL – from health benefits to controlling food cravings. Find Web sites that can give you further help and information on all things low GL. With so much misinformation out there, we trawled the net carefully to find sites where you can trust the contents. Uncover ten savvy food swaps to keep the GL down.

Chapter 14

Ten Reasons for Eating the Low-GL Way

. . . .

In This Chapter

▶ Looking at why low-GL makes sense

▶ Enjoying the low-GL benefits for mind, body, and soul

. . . .

Many eating plans are put together purely to achieve weight loss, but you can experience more than just another short-lived promise when you adopt the Glycaemic Load (GL) Diet. Quick-fix eating plans come and go, and all too often they simply offer rapid, short-term, unsustainable weight loss at the expense of nutritional balance.

The GL Diet is far more than a weight-loss plan. The GL Diet can be part of a healthier, happier lifestyle. In this chapter we give you ten major reasons why a low-GL eating plan is the way forward for both weight control and overall health.

Stabilise Your Blood Sugars

When you eat high-glycaemic foods you experience a rapid increase or a *spike* in glucose (blood sugar). This rise prompts your body to produce *insulin* (a powerful hormone). Insulin flushes the glucose from your bloodstream into your liver and muscles, which store the glucose for later use as energy.

If you constantly eat foods that produce glucose, then you have a continual oversupply in your blood. When your liver and muscles can't store any more, they send the glucose to your fat cells – which expand rapidly! You need to expend energy to use up the stored glucose, but, let's face it, the marathon runners amongst us are in the minority.

Following the glucose spike after eating high-glycaemic foods comes the inevitable rapid fall in blood sugars, which prompts you to redress the balance by eating even more high-glycaemic foods. The cycle is vicious.

Eating low-GL foods means that your blood sugars remain stable because low-GL foods release a steady stream of glucose into the blood rather than a short, sharp glucose rush that you get when you eat high-GL foods. A steady drip-feed of glucose means stable blood sugars and fewer spikes and falls.

Get a Handle on Your Food Cravings

Most people feel an overwhelming need to eat in the middle of the morning or the afternoon. All too often, the only food that can satisfy your craving is something sweet or salty and loaded with fat – in other words, high-GL foods. The fall that follows the spike in blood sugars after you've eaten high-GL foods is the point when food cravings occur most often. Eating more high-glycaemic foods starts the blood sugar roller-coaster all over again.

Choosing low-GL foods at meal and snack times means that the blood sugar roller-coaster stops in its tracks. When you stop the dramatic rise and fall of your blood sugar levels, your cravings for sweet or fatty foods stop, too. Of course, you'll probably fancy some chocolate or your favourite sweet treat occasionally, and you can still enjoy those foods, some of the time. Eating the GL-way puts you back in control of *when* you choose to indulge.

Control Your Weight

You don't need to be a mathematician, or even a dietitian, to work out that if you eat fewer high-calorie, high-fat, high-sugar foods, your overall calorie or energy intake reduces. Cutting down on these types of foods is the fundamental requirement for weight loss.

You can reduce the amount of sugar in your blood by eating the low-GL way, and you can increase your activity levels to burn fat – the most effective way to lose weight and maintain that loss forever.

Level Your Moods

When you eat high-GL foods and your blood sugars go up and down like a yo-yo, so too does your mood. Your brain is your control centre – if your brain is starved of energy, the rest of your body stops working. If one minute your brain has excess energy from high-GL food, and the next minute you have an energy slump, you and everyone around you will feel the effect – your bad mood!

When you're low on fuel you get tetchy, irritable, and short-tempered. Many studies show that your *cognitive performance* (how you think and concentrate) is adversely affected when fuel supplies are low (when you're hungry). Ensuring that your brain has a steady and consistent supply of energy is vital.

Following the low-GL plan is all about eating more foods that drip-feed energy, keeping your blood sugars stable, keeping you level-headed, and keeping everyone around you happy.

Balance Your Hormones

Regularly eating high-glycaemic foods means that the hormone *insulin* (your system for controlling blood sugars) is working in overdrive. Making hormones and putting them to work is no mean feat and takes a lot of energy and resources. Your *endocrine system* (the system that controls your hormones) is involved in just about every aspect of your wellbeing. Your emotional, physical, mental, and even your sexual wellbeing relies on hormones to stimulate, mediate, and control chemical reactions that keep everything in harmony.

If your insulin is working in overdrive, some of your other hormones are likely to suffer as a result. Eating low-GL foods really can help to balance your hormones because their slow release into your system stabilises your blood sugars and enables insulin to work normally.

No Food Is Banned

Imagine a healthy eating plan where nothing, let alone an entire food group, is banned. How refreshing! Eating healthily means getting a better *balance* of foods in your diet to minimise the risk of disease, and does not put a complete ban on certain foods. A great reason to eat the low-GL way is that you don't have to ban anything.

If you know that a food is high-GL, you can make an informed choice about how you want to handle it. With a high-GL food you can:

- Eat a little less of it
- Eat it a little less often
- Mix and match it with other low-GL foods to reduce the overall glycaemic effect (see Chapter 11)
- Cook it in a way that reduces its glycaemic effect

Low-GL Is the Full Story

The Glycaemic Index (GI) Diet was a truly fantastic break-through and helped people realise that certain carbohydrates are more beneficial than others. But GI gives only half the story.

The Glycaemic Load Diet takes into account the rate of release and effect the carbohydrate in a food has on blood sugar. However, GL leaps ahead of GI and also considers the average portion sizes you actually eat at a meal, and how many carbs are in those portions. GL is much more accurate than GI alone, and more helpful in guiding you towards everyday healthy food choices. GL is the final part of the carbohydrate jigsaw.

Anyone Can Do It

Any good eating plan not only needs to provide you with the essential nutrients you need to be healthy, but also needs to be enjoyable. Try enjoying or staying healthy on the Cabbage Soup diet!

The GL Diet is both healthy and enjoyable. GL isn't simply another passing fad or restrictive quick-fix diet. GL is a way of eating that's safe and suitable for adults and children alike. You don't need to take vitamins and mineral supplements as you do with some diet regimes.

You don't need to want to lose weight to enjoy a low-GL way of life. The GL Diet has real potential benefits for people with heart disease, diabetes, and syndrome X (a collection of symptoms that increases the risk of heart disease and diabetes). The GL Diet can also help women suffering from pre-menstrual syndrome (PMS), polycystic ovarian syndrome (PCOS), and the menopause. Head to Chapter 13 for more about the medical benefits of the GL Diet.

Most fruits, beans, nuts, seeds, and vegetables are naturally low-GL, so the GL Diet is perfect for vegetarians.

Clear Labelling

Reading a food label can give you lots of really useful information but only if you know what to look for. We feel strongly that consumers need a clear, easily understandable label to help with choosing healthy foods. Australians and South Africans use the 'G logo' to help identify low-glycaemic foods (refer to Chapter 4). In the UK, some major food retailers now recognise the validity of the low-glycaemic message and provide guidance on food labels. Food labels stating 'low or medium GL' can help you choose a lower glycaemic food within a category of foods, such as picking out the lowest loaf from a selection of breads.

Improve Your Health

The World Cancer Research Fund estimates that eating five portions of fruit and vegetables a day could prevent 20 per cent of deaths from chronic diseases worldwide.

Antioxidant vitamins and minerals found in fruit and vegetables help protect against the *free radicals* (unstable compounds) that damage our genetic material and cause cancer.

Shockingly, some weight-loss plans advocate restricting your intake of fruits and vegetables. The GL Diet positively encourages eating most types of fruit and veg. Take a look at the Cheat Sheet in the front of this book for a list of seasonal low-GL fruit and veg.

Too much saturated and trans fats in your diet can send your blood cholesterol levels soaring. Any eating plan that advises freely eating foods laden with these unhealthy fats is neither safe nor acceptable. The GL way of eating recommends eating foods containing saturated fats sparingly, as a treat. In general, use unsaturated fats in your GL plan, which helps protect against heart disease.

Chapter 15

Ten Best GL Web Sites

●●●

In This Chapter

▶ Finding trustworthy up-to-date information about GL

▶ Checking out the GL of all your favourite foods

▶ Learning more about carbohydrates

▶ Discovering new ways to use low-GL foods

●●●

*T*he Glycaemic Load (GL) is a new and exciting field of nutrition and you can find more and more GL research as each day passes. But how do you know where to go for sound advice that you can trust? With so many sources of advice, especially on the Internet, you can find yourself struggling in an ocean of information – even some misinformation.

In this chapter we show you reliable Web sites dedicated to GL, accurate information about carbs, and ideas for low-GL recipes that really work. Click your mouse to get Web surfing!

American Journal of Clinical Nutrition

www.ajcn.org/cgi/content/full/76/1/5

This link takes you to one of the most important original research articles in the field of GI and GL, and it's fascinating to see the science behind the GL story. The article is well-written, and not too technical. The *American Journal of Clinical Nutrition* is a peer-reviewed scientific journal, which means that you can trust that the research was carried out to the highest standards. Best of all, the appendix contains a table listing the GL for typical serving sizes of over 750 foods.

The article also has links to back issues of the journal with other classic studies (including the article on the Glycaemic Load by Walter Willett mentioned in Chapter 2).

The British Meat Education Service

www.bmesonline.org.uk

The British Meat Education Service (BMES) provides trustworthy information about the safety and nutrition of meat. We chose the site for the ideas it offers on healthy, tasty, low-GL meat dishes. Go to the recipes section and you can access a wealth of suggestions from Deviled Lamb Cutlets to Black Bean Roast Beef. The dishes are displayed in tempting full-colour photos for you to drool over.

You can also link to the BMES's consumer Web site at www.meatmatters.com. From here you can select more recipes, including an option to pick a recipe based on how much time you have available to cook.

 You can peruse recipes from the Meat Matters Web site by adding an ingredient of your choice. Being dedicated low-GL fans, we chose beans. Bingo – we found 29 recipes combining meat and beans. Lamb shanks with cannelloni beans, coming up!

British Nutrition Foundation

www.nutrition.org.uk

The British Nutrition Foundation is a charity offering sound nutritional information and advice to scientists as well as the public. The Web site contains all the key information on basic nutrition, plus advice about nutrition through the stages of life, and the connection between health and nutrition. We like the 'Food Commodities' section where you can browse to find out more about the nutritional value of your favourite low-GL foods.

The British Nutrition Foundation's Web site acts as a gateway into a whole world of other informative nutrition-related sites. Just go to the links page for more sites of interest – the world is your oyster.

Diabetes UK

www.diabetes.org.uk

Diabetes UK is a charity for people with diabetes (the name gives you a clue). The dietary advice section is called 'Eating Well' and applies to most people, diabetic or not. You'll find great practical tips for meal planning, choosing snacks, eating out, and weight management, as well as special diabetes-related topics, such as blood sugar control and what to eat if you're unwell.

You could spend a whole day just cruising around the site for sound nutritional information but we like the way you can easily find what you want when you're in a hurry. Check out the alphabetical information centre covering all areas of diabetes care. For instance, go to 'S' and you get nutritional information on salt, sweeteners, and supplements. Go to 'D' and you get access to the whole field of 'diet and diabetes' side by side with drinking and driving (but not together we hope!).

Diet Freedom

www.dietfreedom.co.uk

This site is perfect if you want to use the low-GL way of eating to help you lose weight. You'll find a fantastic review of the science behind GL, and wonderful tried and tested recipes. We love the online forum discussion for sharing tips and information with other people losing weight the GL-way. In fact, we love this idea so much so that Nigel is now the consultant dietitian for the site.

Food Standards Agency

www.eatwell.gov.uk

The Food Standards Agency (FSA) provides advice and information to the public and to the Government on all aspects of nutrition and diet. The FSA also aims to protect consumers by effective food standards enforcement and monitoring.

The FSA's Web site covers aspects of food safety, technology, hygiene, and nutrition. We particularly like the healthy diet section with 'Nutrition Essentials'. For instance, select their section on pulses, beans, and nuts, and you get the comprehensive lowdown – from what they are, to how to cook them, store them, and use them in recipes.

GI News

www.ginews.blogspot.com

GI News is a free monthly online newsletter billed as the 'official news site for the glycemic index'. Produced by the Glycemic Index Online, the site is a treasure trove of bang up-to-date information on all things GI and GL. You can read research from around the world, news briefs from the previous month, and updates on GL values. GI News also provides a recipe of the month and a GL food of the month to stimulate your adventurous side. You can access all the archived back issues of the newsletter and immerse yourself in GL heaven. You'll find useful information on this site, whether you're completely new to GL or a seasoned old hand.

The Glycemic Index OnLine

www.glycemicindex.com

This GI Web site is run by the University of Sydney. The site is easy to navigate and packed with a wealth of authoritative and comprehensive information on both GI and GL. You can read about the latest studies in a consumer friendly way, and scan reviews of all the latest books on GI and GL.

From the side bar on the left-hand side of the site, you can access a huge database of foods, the 'GI database'. You can either enter a food name to get the GL per serving or you can search for foods with a specified GL – for example, 'all breads with a GL < 10'. Wonderful stuff! You can even view a selection of manufactured products recently analysed for GL. Some of the foods tested are uniquely Australian but many foods overlap with UK and US foods.

Just Eat More (fruit & veg)

www.5aday.nhs.uk

Just Eat More (fruit & veg) is a wonderful, user-friendly Web site run by the Department of Health to promote – you've guessed it – your low-GL friends, fruit and vegetables. The section called 'About 5 a Day' contains all the 'need to know' information about why fruit and vegetables are a key to a healthier lifestyle, and what counts as a portion. The site has lots of tasty trivia about fruit and vegetables, smoothie recipes, and easy meals to try. You'll also find a wonderful section on 'makeovers' for vegetables aiming to make them more attractive (who'd have thought that cauliflower could become cooliflower?). Other fun sections include a downloadable wall chart guaranteed to boost your children's fruit and veg intake, and an interactive sumo smoothie game for teenagers and the young at heart.

This site will really inspire you to eat more low-GL fruit and vegetables.

The Sea Fish Industry Authority (Seafish)

www.seafish.org

Seafish works across all sectors of the UK seafood industry to promote good quality fish, and sustainable fishing. The Web site is a wealth of useful information – if you like fish! Go to the 'On Plate' menu bar for a fascinating and practical guide to buying fresh fish, plus sections on the nutrition of fish.

You'll also find a really useful guide of recommended fish restaurants, pubs, and cafes where you can try out the eating out suggestions in Chapter 5.

The site is packed with ideas for recipes. You can find everything from starters to quick snacks to dishes for entertaining. We especially liked the look of the aromatic mackerel with chickpeas. Dive in and take a look for yourself.

Chapter 16

Ten GL-Savvy Food Swaps

*S*ome diets ban your favourite everyday foods. How mean! Aside from being impractical and inconvenient, this ban is one of the main reasons that so many diets fail because your human nature means that if you're told you can't have something, you tend to want it even more!

The nice thing about eating the low-glycaemic-load way is that no foods are completely forbidden. However, some foods are lower-GL and better for you than others. This chapter shows you that simple, savvy food swaps can really contribute to keeping your GL consumption low. And you can have your chocolate and eat it too!

Getting Your Oats

Boxed breakfast cereals are not always as healthy as they may appear. Some cereals are loaded with salt and sugar, and many are likely to send your blood sugars roller-coasting – not the best start to your low-GL day. But, don't despair: A super quick, simple cereal that ticks all the boxes for health is good old-fashioned porridge oats.

Oats are one of the lowest GL cereals around. A breakfast made with 45 grams of oats with 220 millilitres of skimmed milk takes just 3 minutes to cook in the microwave, so oats are ideal when you're breakfasting in a hurry. If you want to add some sweetness to your porridge, a few chopped, soft, dried apricots do the trick and add even more fibre to your breakfast.

If you don't fancy a hot breakfast in the summer, check out Chapter 6 for our recipe for fast muesli, which also has heaps of other delicious breakfasts to get your day off to a great low-GL start.

Instant hot oat cereals can have a lot of added sugar and are more processed than simple porridge, so stick to the traditional oats.

Sussing Out Sugar

Too much sugar is bad news for your low-GL diet, not to mention your dental health. Try to avoid refined, added sugar as much as possible. The good news is that avoiding sugar doesn't mean you must avoid sweet foods altogether. One alternative is to use artificial sweeteners, but sweeteners can sometimes leave a chemical aftertaste and not all are suitable for cooking. Another alternative to sugar is natural fruit sugar or *fructose*. Fructose looks like sugar, tastes like sugar (in fact, fructose is about one third sweeter than sugar), and most importantly has a less dramatic *glycaemic response* (how quickly the sugar enters the bloodstream – refer to Chapter 2) than regular table sugar or sucrose.

If you want to try fructose for sweetening your coffee, or you want to use it in cooking, check the label on the fructose for quantities and instructions.

Another alternative to sugar is honey. Honey has a moderate GL, so a spoonful here and there won't hurt. Eating your honey with a low-GL food such as oats further reduces the honey's impact on your blood sugars. Head to Chapter 11 for more on food combining to reduce GL.

Pondering Potatoes

Unlike on fussy diets, indulging in some types of potato is just fine and dandy on a low-GL plan. The smaller baby potatoes have a lower GL than large, white, floury varieties. Having a couple of small new potatoes with your evening meal or as a potato salad doesn't have an adverse effect on your blood sugars.

You can eat baked potatoes on a low-GL diet, but instead of the traditional white potato try baking a sweet potato. Sweet potatoes are much quicker to cook in the oven or the microwave, and are delicious with a little butter and black pepper, or some cottage cheese.

As well as being a good source of vitamin C, the bright orange flesh of the sweet potato contains large amounts of beta carotene and vitamin E, which are protective antioxidant vitamins that help to protect your body and reduce damage to your cells.

Sweet potatoes make fantastic mash – head to Chapter 8 for a tasty recipe.

Checking Your Chocolate

If in the past 'diet = no chocolate' was your downfall then do we have great news for you! You *can* eat chocolate on a low-GL diet.

Most chocolate is fattening because it contains large amounts of fat and sugar but the cocoa bean itself is not fattening. A rush of sugar results in a spike (quick rise) and the subsequent plummet of blood sugars and that means that you crave more of the same food. These blood sugar peaks and troughs can lead you to sometimes munch your way through a whole bar of chocolate when you only meant to have one piece. But remember – that's only true for most chocolate!

Chocolate with a high percentage of cocoa solids (at least 70 per cent and ideally 85 per cent) contains much less fat and sugar than regular chocolate, which means better control of your blood sugars and therefore less chance of overindulging.

Dark chocolate is also a rich source of antioxidants known as *flavonols*, which also occur in fruits, red wine, and tea. Flavonols are believed to protect against heart disease, cancer, and high blood pressure.

High cocoa solid chocolate has a much richer flavour than regular chocolate so you find that a couple of pieces is enough to satisfy your craving.

Getting Nutty for Savoury Snacks

If you enjoy settling down with a bowl full of salty potato crisps, what treats can you have on the GL Diet?

Apart from making a huge and unwelcome contribution to your daily salt intake (Chapter 3 has the low-down on salt), potato crisps are a GL nightmare. Crisps are made from large floury potatoes that are then deep-fried, which makes the starches much easier to absorb into the blood.

The perfect alternative savoury snack is a handful (about 30 grams) of unsalted nuts. A small portion of unsalted peanuts reduces hunger pangs (unless you're allergic to them, of course!), and a small portion of almonds or walnuts can even help lower cholesterol levels.

Although the oils in nuts are healthy unsaturated oils, nuts are high in calories, so stick to a 30-gram portion (a small handful).

Another good alternative to potato crisps is some toasted mixed seeds such as sunflower, sesame, and pumpkin seeds. They have a lovely nutty flavour when toasted in a dry pan for a few minutes and are loaded with healthy essential fatty acids and fibre. Chapter 10 has suggestions for handy snacks in a bag using nuts and toasted seeds.

Going Crackers for Oatcakes

Can't imagine cheese and biscuits without the biscuits? You don't have to.

Many varieties of wheat-based crackers have a high-GL, which sets off that old blood sugar roller coaster. Rye crackers and oat cakes are much better choices. Spread a little hummus, peanut butter, or eat with a small piece (matchbox size) of cheese and you've created a great low-GL snack. Add some salad or a bowl of soup and bingo! You've got yourself a perfect lunch.

Chapters 7 and 10 are chock-full of lunch box and snack ideas.

Toning Down the Tipple

Most people enjoy a social drink every now and then, and nothing's wrong with that. In fact, evidence suggests that a moderate alcohol intake could be beneficial to your health. *Moderate* being the key word. Too much of a good thing is bad news for your waistline and, in the case of alcohol, for a whole host of other bits, such as your liver! In terms of GL, the drinks to avoid are the sugar-laden alcopops, liqueurs, fortified wines and sherries, and sweet cider. Your best options are spirits with diet or slimline mixers. Choose red wine over white, or if you dislike red wine, choose dry white wine over sweet. If you prefer a beer, choose a brand with a low-carbohydrate option. Lucky that the low-carb craze left us consumers with some good things!

Check out Chapter 5 for more on choosing alcoholic drinks and the recommended safe drinking limits.

Passing the Pasta

Treat pasta as a side dish, rather than the main part of your meal and it's fine to eat on a low-GL diet. (Refer to Chapter 14 to find out how GL helps you get a more accurate picture of what happens to your blood sugars when you eat pasta.)

Pasta has a moderate GL but what you eat with it and how you cook your pasta lessens its effect on blood sugars. Sauces made from vegetables such as tomatoes, or sauces combined with lean proteins such as fish and chicken or beans, and even a little sprinkle of parmesan all help to slow the rise in blood sugars caused by eating your linguini or fettuccine. Most important is to cook your pasta the Italian way – *al dente*, or firm to the bite. Overcooked pasta has a much higher GL than pasta cooked just right, so check labels for exact cooking times.

Push the GL from pasta even lower by mixing pasta and pulses (beans or lentils) 50/50. Beans such as butter beans, chickpeas, and aduki beans have a low GL and help to lower the GL of the meal. Buy canned beans to avoid hours of soaking and boiling.

Take a look at Chapter 8 for delicious recipes using pasta.

Replacing Rice

As a very general rule wild rice or long grain brown rice varieties such as brown Basmati rice tend to be slightly lower in GL than the short grain white varieties.

Rice can be high in GL because of the type of starch it contains. Amylose is the tiny compound that joins up to form a grain of rice. The more amylose rice contains, the lower the GL. However, amylose doesn't appear on labels so you don't know how much is in your rice. Also, the exact amylose content varies from one crop of rice to another of the same rice anyway, so even if the amylase content did appear on a label it would probably be inaccurate.

When it comes to rice, like pasta, mix your wild or basmati rice with pulses such as lentils to lower the GL. Alternatively, you can use bulgur wheat, couscous, or quinoa instead of rice. These grains all have a moderate GL and are fine when served in small portions. Chapter 8 gives plenty of suggestions for combining rice with other grains.

Picking through the Bread Basket

Wholemeal breads have almost the same high GL as white, refined bread, and neither is great for your low-GL lifestyle. Don't worry though; you can find some delicious bread that fits the bill just fine. If you're lucky enough to have a good bakery near you, experiment with dark rye or pumpernickel breads, and both are great low-GL choices. Pre-sliced packaged barley and sunflower breads or soya and linseed breads are also good choices from the supermarket.

If you're stuck with a limited choice of bread at a restaurant or in the supermarket, the golden rule is to pick the grainiest, seediest bread you can – the bread with the most 'bits'. The seeds and grains slow the rollercoaster blood sugar effect of the rest of the bread. However, your best practice is to stick to including just a small amount of bread in your diet – always.

Chapter 10 has plenty of ideas for tasty snacks on toast.

Appendix

A–Z List of Low-GL Foods

*T*his A–Z list is an extension of the information you can find in the shopping guide in Chapter 4.

GL testing is developing all the time, but you can find regularly updated food lists on www.dietfreedom.co.uk.

The foods included in these lists have a GL of 10 or less, making them a low-GL food when you eat them in the portions size stated. We focus mainly on carbohydrate foods and a few miscellaneous items that you may find useful as low-GL sweet treats. We haven't included fruits, vegetables, dairy foods, or fats and oils, and you won't find protein foods such as meat, fish, poultry, and pulses (beans and lentils) either. Although some of these foods contain carbohydrate, they have a negligible effect on blood sugars, so providing you follow the general healthy eating principles we discuss in Chapters 3 and 12 you'll be doing just fine.

The main focus of the GL Diet is to reduce the roller-coaster effect on your blood sugars by choosing more low-GL foods. Carbs have a big effect on your blood sugars, so use this list to help you keep on track.

If a food is normally eaten cooked, assume the GL refers to a cooked portion.

Grains and cereals
- Buckwheat (100g)
- Bulgar wheat (100g)
- Cous cous (100g)
- Muesli (no added sugar) (30g)
- Oat bran (10g)
- Porridge oats (steel cut) (30g dry weight)

- Quinoa (30g dry weight)
- Rice bran (30g)
- Rye (whole) (30g dry weight)
- Semolina (100g)
- Wheat (whole) (30g)

Starchy staples

- Brown rice (75g)
- Potatoes (Baby new) (80g)
- Rice noodles (100g)
- Soba (buckwheat) noodles (100g)
- Spaghetti, white (100g)
- Spaghetti, wholemeal (100g)
- Sweet potatoes (80g)
- Wild rice (75g)

Breads and crackers

- Dark rye bread (30g)
- Oat bran and honey bread (30g)
- Oat cakes (30g)
- Pumpernickel bread (30g)
- Rye crackers (30g)
- Sourdough bread (30g)
- Soya and linseed bread (30g)
- Spelt multigrain bread (30g)
- Sunflower and barley bread (30g)
- Wholegrain bread (30g)
- Wholemeal pitta bread (30g)
- Wholemeal rye bread (30g)

Sweets and treats

- Chocolate (High cocoa solid) (20g)
- Fructose (10g)
- Honey (25g)
- Ice cream (vanilla) (50g)
- Popcorn (20g)

Index

Notes

FOR DUMMIES®

Do Anything. Just Add Dummies

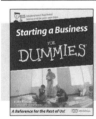
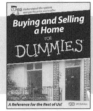
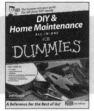
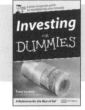
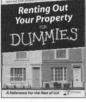
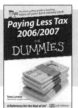
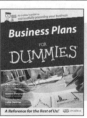
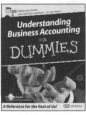
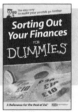

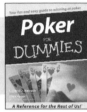
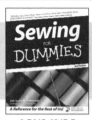
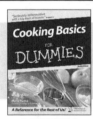
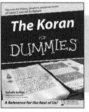
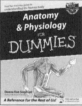
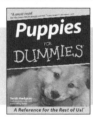
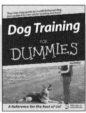
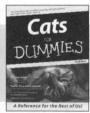

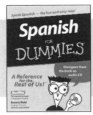
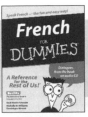
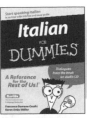
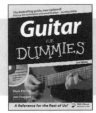
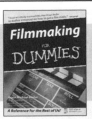
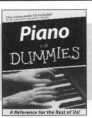
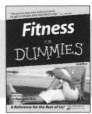
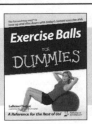
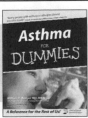

FOR DUMMIES

INTERNET

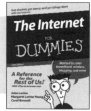

0-7645-8996-2

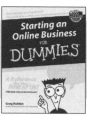

0-7645-8334-4

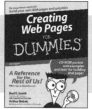

0-7645-7327-6

Also available:

eBay.co.uk
For Dummies
(0-7645-7059-5)

Dreamweaver 8
For Dummies
(0-7645-9649-7)

Web Design
For Dummies
(0-471-78117-7)

Everyday Internet
All-in-One Desk
Reference
For Dummies
(0-7645-8875-3)

Creating Web Pages
All-in-One Desk
Reference
For Dummies
(0-7645-4345-8)

DIGITAL MEDIA

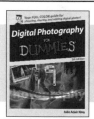

0-7645-9802-3

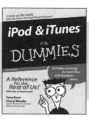

0-471-74739-4

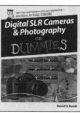

0-7645-9803-1

Also available:

Digital Photos,
Movies, & Music
GigaBook
For Dummies
(0-7645-7414-0)

Photoshop CS2
For Dummies
(0-7645-9571-7)

Podcasting
For Dummies
(0-471-74898-6)

Blogging
For Dummies
(0-471-77084-1)

Digital Photography
all in one desk
reference
For Dummies
(0-7645-7328-4)

Windows XP Digital
Music For Dummies
(0-7645-7599-6)

COMPUTER BASICS

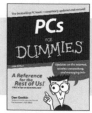

0-7645-8958-X

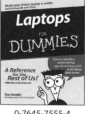

0-7645-7555-4

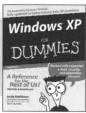

0-7645-7326-8

Also available:

Office XP 9 in 1
Desk Reference
For Dummies
(0-7645-0819-9)

PCs All-in-One Desk
Reference
For Dummies
(0-471-77082-5)

Pocket PC For
Dummies
(0-7645-1640-X)

Upgrading & Fixing
PCs For Dummies
(0-7645-1665-5)

Windows XP All-in-
One Desk Reference
For Dummies
(0-7645-7463-9)

Macs For Dummies
(0-7645-5656-8)

8322_p4